THE ELEMENTS OF TAI CHI

Paul Crompton has studied Tai Chi and other martial arts for over twenty years and has been a teacher of Tai Chi for about fifteen years. He founded the *Karate and Oriental Arts* magazine in 1966 and has published seventy books on the different martial arts as well as completing three videos on Tai Chi, Karate and Kung Fu.

The *Elements Of* is a series designed to present high quality introductions to a broad range of essential subjects.

The books are commissioned specifically from experts in their fields. They provide readable and often unique views of the various topics covered, and are therefore of interest both to those who have some knowledge of the subject, as well as those who are approaching it for the first time.

Many of these concise yet comprehensive books have practical suggestions and exercises which allow personal experience as well as theoretical understanding, and offer a valuable source of information on many important themes.

THE ELEMENTS OF
TAI CHI

Paul Crompton

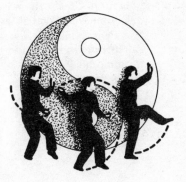

ELEMENT BOOKS

First published in Great Britain in 1990 by
Element Books Limited
Longmead, Shaftesbury, Dorset

Cover Design by Max Fairbrother
Illustrations by Pauline Howcroft
Typeset by Selectmove, London
Printed and bound in Great Britain by
Billings Ltd, Hylton Road, Worcester

British Library Cataloguing in Publication Data
Crompton, Paul
The elements of Tai Chi.
1. T'ai chi ch'uan
I. Title
796.8155
ISBN 1–85230–157–0

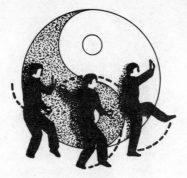

CONTENTS

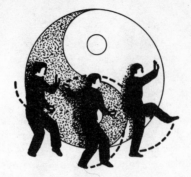

INTRODUCTION

Moving slowly, under the trees, breathing, it seems, in time with a gentle breeze; merging with Nature itself in a healing rhythm. Head, shoulders, arms, trunk, legs and feet moving as one; continuously, smoothly and restfully; as if swimming into a new, all-pervading element; a different time, a different space . . .

Poor words, but an attempt to convey the experience of performing the movements of T'ai Chi Ch'uan, the Chinese art of soft and gentle exercise. Western usage has reduced the full expression to Tai Chi, and this abbreviation will be used in the book. The art is said to be the child of Taoist teachings, but its origin has disappeared into the mists of the past. To describe this art of movement is a little like trying to describe music with words; destined to fail perhaps, but interesting to attempt for all that.

The history of Taoism itself throws some light on the history of Tai Chi, for they both demonstrate two levels of understanding on the part of those who followed them in the past and who follow them today. The earliest and deeper level of Taoism taught a way of understanding man and his relationship with the universe by indicating that any attempt by man to 'do' or to interfere with the natural order of things was an error, based on ignorance of the workings of the Tao. The Tao, the Way of Heaven, was displayed in the natural order of things, and man could only perceive this natural order by becoming one with it; not by analysing and manipulating it. Those who followed the Taoist Way were referred to as Men of Tao. (A close approximation to the pronunciation of 'Tao' is 'Dow' as in the English word 'how'.) The later, degenerated form of Taoist *religion* became mixed with magic, occultism, manipulation of energy, and 'doing';

methods of interfering with the natural order instead of yielding to it.

The purest approach to Tai Chi is essentially an approach to following the earlier form of Taoist philosophy through movement. Tai Chi is sometimes known as meditation in movement. But the art has become contaminated with many other influences, foreign to its nature, which will be explained in this book. The two levels of understanding are clearly not limited to the subject of Tai Chi or Taoism but seem to appear in all human encounters with the traditional Ways.

Tai Chi today is little more than a reminder that at one time people studied and practised it who had real knowledge of the place of man in the universe. This is not a harsh statement, in my view, but simply a fact. Throughout Chinese history, eminent and obscure Taoists influenced behaviour and thought at many levels of society. The influence was felt by scholars, farmers, Mongolian khans and emperors. But that time has gone, the source has gone, and now we have a situation in which here and there in different parts of the world there are some respected Taoists and Tai Chi masters, but the entire context into which Taoism was born and flourished, and into which Tai Chi was introduced, no longer exists. This Chinese art of movement is like a finger pointing at the moon.

There are several different threads running through this book, which represent different points of view. One comes from my own experience of over twenty years of studying Tai Chi and other approaches to the inner life of mankind. Another is taken from the writings and experiences of Tai Chi teachers, writers and students. A third emerges from the words of scholars such as Professor Fung Yu-lan, author of *A Short History of Chinese Philosophy*,[1] which I recommend to all students of Tai Chi who wish to broaden their background knowledge. In the book the author points out that Chinese philosophy is expressed in the form of 'suggestive' aphorisms. Their brevity is meant to inspire 'reflective thinking' and contrasts with the 'articulate' pronouncements of western philosophy, which aim to be as exact and explicit as possible. This contrast between suggestion and articulate expression has spread into the study and teaching of Tai Chi in a manner which causes confusion. One finds in the writings of some Tai Chi teachers, especially modern ones, a mixture of fact, misinformation, wisdom, fantasy and poetic imagery. It is hoped that this book will help to make the contents of that mind-boggling cocktail a little clearer.

The suggestive aphorisms of the Taoist philosophy are meant to evoke a mood in which the movements of Tai Chi are performed. Through western influences there has been an influx of attempted *articulate suggestions* – a contradiction in terms. There can be no articulate explanation for the necessary mood. The best known book of Taoist wisdom is the *Tao Te Ching*.[2] The opening lines read: 'The Tao that is expressed in words is not the true Tao.' The whole book creates a mood, an attitude towards life, and the wise sayings which are used in Tai Chi books should be approached in the same way. They are like many sticks of incense of different flavours all burning simultaneously to produce an overall scent. This scent should inform the Tai Chi movements.

So different threads run through this book, producing, it is hoped, a tapestry of Tai Chi such as any student of the art might weave, for himself or herself. For us westerners this is preferable to trying to adopt either the suggestive or articulate approach exclusively, because to do so would be artificial. We need to find our own understanding of Tai Chi.

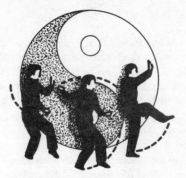

1 · THE HISTORY OF TAI CHI

Chinese people have emigrated and settled in just about every country in the world. This has meant that Chinese culture has taken root everywhere, and this culture includes the art of Tai Chi. Consequently, any history would have to be encyclopaedic if it were to be comprehensive. Secondly, although there are today only three main schools of Tai Chi – Chen, Wu and Yang – there are a number of minor schools and derivatives of the three main ones. Every school or style performs the movements in its own characteristic way, so to document the dozens of variations would also present an impossible task, partly because many of them have not been recorded and the style in some cases has disappeared. Thirdly, it is difficult to separate true accounts of the history of Tai Chi from legend, hearsay and fantasy. These three formidable factors make the task of giving even an accurate, potted history quite a problem for any writer. So I present here a selection of what I have been able to ascertain, and apologise in advance for any omissions or seeming errors to Tai Chi students and teachers who in the main are very ardent in their beliefs about the lineage and background of their art.

All accounts of the history of Tai Chi make mention of the legendary Chang San-feng. He was a Taoist Immortal; eccentric, playful, over two metres tall, a formidable fighter, always unkempt in appearance and immensely strong. Being an immortal he could have existed at any time, and the many accounts of his life and references to him bear this out. A hundred years before the Ming dynasty, in the 13th century, he

1

is written about as the friend of a well-known figure, Liu Ping-chung (1216–74) a Ch'an monk connected with Kubilai Khan. In the Sung dynasty (960–1279) Chang San-feng appears from time to time. From 1368 to 1398 he is supposed to have travelled in Szechwan. During his travels he stayed with a certain family and used to sit in meditation in their garden. One day he planted some branches of a plum tree in the ground as he sat and they immediately burst into blossom. Later still he was glimpsed in Shantung province riding on the back of a flying crane. In 1459 he was made a saint by Emperor Ying-tsun. The name of Immortal Penetrating Mystery And Revealing Transformation was conferred upon him. Oblivious to imperial favours, Chang continued to roam, apparently without any outside aims, but always nourishing the inner process of his own continuing immortality. One of the places he stayed in, the Wu-tang peak district in northern Hopei, was to become famous in Tai Chi history. It was already an abode of Taoist hermits and home of the god of War, Hsuan-lang, who had a shrine built there in his honour. In the days before the Sung dynasty, his title had been god of the North.

During the Yung-lo period a high commissioner was sent by the emperor to search the Wu-tang peak district to try to find Chang. For a thirteen year period, between 1407 and 1423, presumably taking three years off to rest, the luckless high commissioner searched, but never found his quarry. The explanation given by scholars in some cases for the protracted search for Chang is that emperors and men in high places were eager to be associated with him and to heap honours upon him, because such association would help them to bask in Chang's glory. This eagerness for reflected glory is also the reason offered for the connection which has been made between Chang and the origins of Tai Chi. The external, hard styles of Chinese martial arts had been associated with the founder of the Ch'an Buddhist sect, Bodhidharma, and it was felt that the internal style of Tai Chi needed a founder of equal stature – to wit, Chang San-feng. In fact, for all his greatness, Bodhidharma was a mere mortal . . .

The earliest known mention of Chang San-feng as a martial artist is found in the biography of a well known boxing master of the time, Chang Sung-ch'i, who lived in the 16th century, in Ning-po. (The word 'boxing' translates the Chinese word 'ch'uan', though the latter means more than merely fighting with the fists; rather the whole study, training and philosophy of martial arts ways.) Chang Sung-ch'i said that he had been taught his art by an alchemist called Chang San-feng who lived as a hermit on the Wu-tang peaks. The alchemist had learned in his turn from the Dark Emperor, during a very graphic dream. Later, he had used the techniques imparted to him in this strange way to defeat some one hundred brigands. The name given to the fighting methods which Chang Sung-ch'i used is not Tai Chi, as one might expect, but 'nei-chia' or 'internal/esoteric school'. Some writers have maintained that Nei Chia and Tai Chi are the same but the more impartial point out that this is a mistake. Part of the evidence for refuting this link comes from a stone epitaph for a certain Wang Cheng-nan, in the 17th century, on which it is shown that Chang passed on his methods of fighting from teacher to teacher until it reached Wang Cheng-nan himself. Wang Cheng-nan's style of boxing was called Nei Chia. From that time the Wu-tang peak district has been associated with Nei Chia, internal style and because of the (probably erroneous) connection made between Nei Chia and Tai Chi, the district has also been linked with Tai Chi. The movements of the two arts differ, and there are no references to or uses of the words Tai Chi in writings on Nei Chia.

So, if Chang San-feng lived at all, he was probably connected to Nei Chia alone. Authorities on the Ming period such as Anna Seidel, a doctor of Chinese history, and teachers of Tai Chi such as Dr Tseng Ju-pai (Chiu Yen) propose that intentional or unintentional confusion of names was the cause of the problem. There were two men with similar names. First there was the Wang Tsung mentioned on the epitaph, who came from Shensi province; second there was a Wang Tsung-yueh of Shansi province who is said to have been the founder of the Chen style of Tai Chi. The Nei Chia school of internal boxing of which Wang Tsung was a member was found in Chekiang province, and the Tai Chi school of Wang Tsung-yueh was in Honan province. Readers will reasonably conclude that we are looking into very murky water here!

In some books on Tai Chi you will find one version of this story and in others the alternative, depending on the author's choice and erudition. People who like to have their history bathed in legend will go for Chang San-feng, and those who like to stick to the facts will discount him or leave him in the air, which is after all his second home!

A second theory about the origins of Tai Chi is that it began during the T'ang dynasty (618–907). It is said that there were four separate schools of martial arts and exercise using similar movements. The founder of the first was a certain man called Hsu Hsun-ping (Hsa Suan-ming) who was a hermit. His style was called the Three Generations and Seven, and it consisted of thirty-seven postures containing the Eight Trigrams in the arm movements and the Five Elements in the leg movements (see Chapter 7). It was said that his style was based on the understanding of the I-Ching.

The second school was called Long Ch'uan or Long Fist/Boxing. The founder of this style of movement was Li Tao-tzu, yet another Immortal. He is supposed to have been very reluctant to speak. When he met anyone his only words to them were 'Good Luck!'. Of the other two schools there is even less to say, except that they were created by Yin Li-hsiang and Cheng Ling-si. The theory goes on to state that Chang San-feng integrated the four schools into one, to make Tai Chi. But none of the schools bore the name Tai Chi nor anything like it, and it is the practice of scholars and teachers to discount this second theory.

A third claim gives the credit for founding Tai Chi to the Wang Tsung-yueh of Shansi mentioned earlier. Like a wandering adventurer of the Wild West he was passing one day through a Chen family village in Honan province between 1736 and 1795. He paused to watch some of the locals training in martial arts and then went on to wash the dust from his lips and put up at the village inn for the night. As a traveller he was an object of respectful curiosity and was soon engaged in conversation. He made some passing remark about the standard of martial arts in the village and this provoked a number of challenges from the Chen villagers. Wang accepted them and trounced them all. His method of fighting was 'soft' or internal, not relying solely on strength and force. This impressed the Chen fraternity and the leaders of the village asked Wang to stay on and teach them. He agreed, and this marked the beginning of the Chen style of Tai Chi in China. This theory though makes no mention of where Wang learned his art, nor from whom. Before continuing the story of the Chen style, a fourth theory of the origins of Tai Chi should be given.

This is the account most favoured by the Chen family descendants, mainly because it gives the inspiration for creating Tai Chi firmly to the Chen family and relies on no outsiders. The founding of Tai Chi according to this theory took place during the Ming dynasty (1368–1654). This tendency of the Chinese to keep things in the family is very characteristic of all their martial arts. Even so, in the case of the Chen family, credit is given to other styles of martial arts upon which the founder, Chen Wang-t'ing, based his creation.

The last two theories are the ones which are most widely held today. Of the two the majority of writers and teachers hold the view that Wang Tsung-yueh was the founder of Tai Chi. Admittedly there were other forms of exercise, of internal arts, of soft, flowing movement, long before Chen or Wang were born. But when it comes to definitions one must draw the line somewhere. The ancient Greeks had fist fights wearing gloves embedded with pieces of sharp metal; fights which were sometimes to the death. But we would hardly call that boxing.

Attempts have been made to push Wang Tsung-yueh out of the picture but an interesting story is told about Yang Lu-ch'an, the founder of Yang style Tai Chi, which helps to retain Wang's image. Yang said that he was a pupil of Ch'en Chang-hsing (1771–1853) of Chen Chia Kou village. Chen had learned from Chiang Fa who in turn learned from Wang. Evidence to support this was found, so it is said, by Wu Yu-seong (1812–1880) a pupil of Yang Lu-ch'an. Wu went to see his brother who lived in Honan province. This meant that he would pass through places not too far from the home of his teacher's teacher, Chen Chang-hsing. He determined to go and pay his respects to the venerable teacher of his teacher. On the way he got into conversation with a local man who told him that another member of the Chen family, Chen Ch'ing-p'ing, was teaching a superior form of Tai Chi. Wu went out of his way a second time in order to see this prodigy. He was allowed to watch the training in progress and was so impressed that he gave up his Yang style for a time and studied the new form of Chen style.

During his stay in the region he met a seller of salt in the Wu Yang district. This man said that he had had a book written by Wang Tsung-yueh and that Wu's brother had bought it from him. Wu hurried to see his brother and asked to read the book – it revealed that Wang Tsung-yueh had indeed taught the Chen family. Wu studied the book deeply, trained with Chen Ch'ing-p'ing and in turn wrote his own book about the art. His first teacher, Yang Lu-ch'an, was sufficiently impressed by it to accept a copy as a present and also to see that his pupils received one each. It appeared from Wang Tsung's preface to his own book that he had for many years been interested in perfecting his technique with the lance, and more importantly that he had lived in Honan province near the Chen family village concerned.

Since 1949 the Chinese have promoted their martial arts on a wide scale and made efforts to bring together histories and genealogies of each art. The genealogy currently presented from mainland China makes no mention of Wang Tsung-yueh or Chiang Fa. Instead, credit for originating Tai Chi is given to Chen Wang-t'ing. This may be due to internal string pulling rather than historical fact, however. In most of the genealogies produced outside China by Chinese writers who hail from pre-revolutionary China, Chen is shown as the pupil of Chiang Fa who in turn was taught by Wang Tsung-yueh. Furthermore, although the above-mentioned Wu Yu-seong is shown in some charts as a pupil of Yang Lu-ch'an, in others he is shown as a pupil of Chen Ch'ing-p'ing. He was in fact a pupil of both. Wu created his own, fully recognised style, the Wu style, and this is probably closer to the Chen than the Yang style.

5

Beginning with Chen Wang-t'ing the better-documented history of Tai Chi can be traced. He studied many martial arts in his youth and handed on to the Chen village the following methods. He combined deep breathing and mental concentration with animal movement exercises to be found in the Chi Kung aspects of Chen style. He studied the theories of Chinese traditional medicine and invented turning, arcing and spiral movements which purported to stimulate the Chi energy running along the acupuncture channels. He introduced movements which alternate between the two extremes of yang, hard, and yin, soft. He also invented the two person Push Hands training exercises (see p.51). The use of the Tai Chi spear, in particular the 'sticking spear' methods (see p.66), was developed by him. Finally, he plunged into explanations and elaborations of theories which dealt with the how and why of Tai Chi. His life ended on a sad note, as far as we can tell. He wrote: 'All the favours bestowed on me are now in vain! Now old and feeble, I am accompanied only by the book of 'Huang Ting'. Life consists of creating actions of boxing when feeling depressed, doing field work when the season comes, and spending leisure time teaching disciples and children so that they can become worthy members of society'.[3] Even so, he laid the foundations of a style that developed, thrived and gave health and enjoyment to thousands.

But not all the new forms of Tai Chi movement invented by Chen Wang-t'ing survived. He passed on seven sets of Tai Chi boxing routines. After only a few generations there were few people who could do the whole syllabus of training. Chen family members could do only the first and second forms of the solo exercise programme, the sticking spear training and the pushing hands. During this time what remained of Chen's work split into two separate parts. Chen Yu-pun created the New Style which did away with the more difficult techniques. Chen Ch'ing-p'ing produced a slower style, which was more compact in its movements. There then existed three styles of Chen family Tai Chi: what remained of the Old Style, the New Style of Chen Yu-pun and the Chen style of Chen Ch'ing-p'ing. Exact dates are not known but the changes occurred sometime during the second half of the nineteenth century.

Wu Yu-seong, who had begun studying Tai Chi with Yang Lu-ch'an and later went to Chen Ch'ing-p'ing, founded his own Wu style, which, as we shall see later, became known as the Old Wu Style. His Tai Chi descendants of note included Hao Wei-chen (Hao Style) and Sun Lu-t'ang (Sun style).

The famous founder of the Yang family style, Yang Lu-ch'an, is said to have gained access to the closely guarded secrets of the Chen family by spying on them from a hidden vantage point and memorising what he had seen. After no less than ten years of this trying to learn on his own he was finally discovered by Chen family members who ordered him to show them what he had achieved. Such was his skill and fidelity to the art that he was accepted as a student; a rare step in those days. He learned the Old Style, but gradually changed it and adapted it as a method of keeping fit rather than as a method of fighting. This modified Chen style was learned by the third son of Yang Lu-ch'an, Yang Chien-hou, who taught it under the name of Middle Style. The third son of Yang Chien-hou, Yang Cheng-fu, studied under his father and he changed the movements into a slow, continuous and graceful style which he called the Big Style.

Readers who have been following this rather tortuous history will appreciate that it is here that something approximating to what we in the West regard as a Taoist spirit enters the art. Up until the coming of the Yang family and even during its promotion of the art, Tai Chi movements varied in speed, in strength and ferocity. They were very much oriented towards fighting. It appears that Yang Cheng-fu was instrumental in bringing the movements into one harmonious tempo and so this raises questions about the historicity of Tai Chi as a Taoist method, and also our western perception of what Taoism is. This will be examined later on.

The Big Style became the basis of most of the Tai Chi that is practised in the West today. It is best known in two solo forms; the Long Form and the Short Form of Cheng Man-ch'ing. Returning to the fate of the Chen style, we find that the remnants of the Old Style were brought to Peking in 1928 by Chen Fake. From then on this branch of the Chen style underwent various changes but still survives and thrives in China today. Notable among the pupils of Chen Fake is Feng Zhiqiang, born in 1926, and Chen Xiaowang, born in 1946. In addition to Cheng Man-ch'ing, notable modern exponents of Yang style were Chen Wei-ming and Tung Ying-chieh.

As far as one can gather, there are two Wu styles in existence today. One is the Old Style of Wu Yu-seong, initially based on the Yang Lu-ch'an and Chen Ch'ing-p'ing styles. The other originated from Wu Chien-ch'uan, a pupil of Ch'uan Yu who had learned from Yang Lu-ch'an. This second style spread to Singapore and is popular there.

This intricate outline of the history of Tai Chi in terms of who taught whom will give the reader some idea of the complexities of the whole subject. If tracing the history within the confines of the three major styles is so difficult, imagine what a pursuit of all the minor styles would be like. Suffice it to say therefore that the Chen style of the art was the original basis for all the existing styles, as far as we know. The information given comes from many sources and it is always possible that mistakes have been made. However, this is the skeleton of the history; what of the flesh? What of the men and women who studied the art and contributed so much to it? What were they looking for? How hard did they study? These are all interesting questions, and a selection of accounts will give more substance to the genealogical bones. One must bear in mind that such accounts are all tinged with imagination, the wish, in some cases, to aggrandise the person concerned and the well known failings of human memory.

Cheng Man-ch'ing, sometimes written Cheng Man-jan, deserves a special place in this chapter because of the wide influence his teachings and writings have had in the West. This influence was partly due to his undoubted skill and understanding but also to the fact that westerners could not wander about in mainland China after the revolution. If they had been able to do so, other eminent masters of other styles would have been found and promoted in western countries and the whole western Tai Chi picture would have been different.

Cheng was born in Chekiang province in 1901. His father died when he was a small child and Cheng was very much influenced by his mother, who taught him poetry and calligraphy. He also attended school near Mount Kuang-lu, and in his spare time he would visit Buddhist temples in the vicinity. Cheng had an extraordinarily good memory and it is said that by the age of nine he had memorised the classics of Confucian teaching. A serious accident occurred when a brick from a wall fell on his head. He fell into a deathly coma for two days. Prognosis was bad and everyone expected him to die, when a martial arts expert appeared on the scene, ascertained that the brick had done the damage and straight away went off into the neighbouring mountains. He returned with some herbs and applied them to the unconscious boy. Cheng recovered consciousness. His brain did not recover completely at first though, and according to Tam Gibbs, a longtime pupil and associate of Cheng's, 'young Cheng had completely lost his memory and was like a vegetable'.

But he slowly recovered and by the age of fourteen he was sufficiently skilled at painting to be able to support his family. His apprenticeship in painting had been unusually swift. His teacher, Wang Hsiang-chan, recognised and encouraged his inborn talents. The gift for painting was echoed in the fields of medicine, calligraphy, classical studies, poetry and martial arts. Before Cheng took up martial arts he suffered from rheumatism, beriberi and tuberculosis; the latter reaching a stage where he coughed up blood. At this time he was in his mid-twenties. He was not expected to survive this illness, which was widespread in China at that time. Then a friend introduced him to Yang Cheng-fu who was already renowned for his Tai Chi skills. Cheng began to study Tai Chi and his health improved. As soon as it did so, he stopped training and his illness came back. Filled with regret at his folly, Cheng began to train again and his health improved until he became quite robust. He wrote: 'I came to see it (Tai Chi) as more important than food or sleep',[4] and from then on he trained daily without fail. Wherever he travelled his skill in painting, his learning and his Tai Chi went with him and brought him admiration, support and students. In Taiwan he established the Shr Jung School of Tai Chi. He died in Taipei on March 26th, 1975.

Cheng's first and eldest student, who became more of a disciple, was T'ung Tsai Liang, born in Hopei province in 1900, one year before his teacher. Liang was with Cheng for twenty years and became a respected teacher in his own right. He assisted Cheng with work at the United Nations in New York and also taught at Boston College, Harvard University, Amherst and other American colleges. Among his Tai Chi classmates were William C.C. Chen and Benjamin Lo, both of whom are well known instructors in the United States. Liang also studied painting, calligraphy and translating, as well as writing commentaries on the classics. American students of these two men include Tam Gibbs, Jonathan Russell, Jerry Kuehl, and Stuart Olave Olsen, to name but a few! They and others have kept the flame of Cheng's Tai Chi burning.

What characterises Cheng's handed-down form of Tai Chi training, as far as one can gather, is its softness, its humanity, and the relative smallness of the movements compared with the large movements of Yang Cheng-fu, his teacher, and Chen Wei-ming. A story current for many years among Chinese martial artists is that Cheng changed what he had learned from Yang and produced his Short Form for the sake of western students whom he initially thought would be unable or unwilling to do the more strenuous Long Form. This is a moot point and provokes animated discussion when raised.

Chinese martial artists are adept at disguising one movement within another to such an extent that beginners are completely baffled. As you become more experienced in martial arts and begin to plough the soil of what you have received you begin to realise the presence of movement within movement. The film of Cheng which is pirated throughout the world gives no hint to an outsider of its latent power. The movements are slow, precise and outwardly innocuous; curative even. But one point worthy of note is the depth of Cheng's stance; that is, the low knee bend, partly concealed by the long light gown he is wearing. Such a deep stance contains power in the legs which can be transmitted to the hand when pushing, or punching. In the same film he is shown pushing several assailants away and resisting being pushed by the same men, all at once, and generally conveying an impression of hidden strength.

The martial arts were given a powerful push West by Cheng. Writer Robert W. Smith[5] studied with Liang, Cheng's first pupil, and later with Cheng himself and he has many tales of the latter dealing with men twice his weight who attacked him and having no trouble in neutralising their attacks. Now there are many students of students of Cheng and Liang. Cheng's own books on Tai Chi have markedly spread his particular message, but once the teacher has gone, it is hard to keep the message clear. My own impression, having met some of his pupils, from Europe, the United States and Singapore, is that there has grown up a tendency to over-stress softness, especially in the area of Push Hands. This underlines the difficulty of good transmission of Tai Chi on a large scale. Unless you can study with an accomplished teacher and pick up a percentage of every aspect of his art you are in danger of going away with one or two, emphasising them, and becoming lop-sided.

Though I am sure that they must exist, I myself have not met a descendant of Cheng's school who seemed free in his or her movements when it came to Push Hands. The search for softness of movement can apparently lead to a kind of tension or hesitation, an unwillingness to risk. This is explained by a remark attributed to Cheng when he was asked why it was that his pupils did not come near him in skill. He said that they had no faith. They had no faith in one of his favourite sayings, that one should 'invest in loss'. This means being willing to lose balance, in order to find it; being willing to yield and so be free.

Wang Pei-sheng of Peking, born in 1910, is a lineal Tai Chi descendant of Ch'uan Yu, who was a pupil of Yang Pan-hou, son of Yang Lu-ch'an. His is one of the Wu styles. Ch'uan Yu was one of a number of bodyguards assigned to a Chinese royal family. He came from Manchuria and began to study with Yang Lu-ch'an. One of the later members of his line was Yang Yu-ting, and Wang Pei-sheng became Yang Yu-ting's student.

Wang's day of Tai Chi is something to think about! He used to rise from bed at three o'clock in the morning and go out into Tianamen Square where he trained alone at the forms and at Tai Chi weapons. This lasted for three hours until six, when the doors of the Grand Temple opened and he went into the rooms which housed the Tai Chi Study

Society. This is now known as the Working People's Cultural Palace. There Wang assisted his teacher in instructing the first Tai Chi class until eight o'clock. At eight a group of elderly and sick people came in and they were taught and encouraged until ten. Finally the more advanced students began their training session which continued for two hours until noon. Wang Pei-sheng followed this regime for three years. It emphasises the effort and devotion which the masters of the art bring to their work.

Yang Cheng-fu, (1883–1936), is the most written-about Tai Chi master of this century in Hong Kong and mainland China. As a child he had no liking for the art and only took it up seriously in his early twenties. On the death of his father his whole attitude changed and he began to try to plumb the depths of Tai Chi. He took up residence in Shanghai and taught martial arts there in a special school, which had been organised by his pupil Chen Wei-ming. Chen Wei-ming was working at the time in the Ching Dynasty History Institute.

During this period, Yang's Tai Chi was said to be very powerful, with fast-kicking techniques. From what we know of the Chen style it seems as though Yang's art still owed a lot to that style's variations in speed, it's power and size of movement. Then Yang began to realise that Tai Chi could do a lot for the treatment of chronic diseases, building up one's health and promoting long life. He started to introduce modifications into what he had been taught and reorganised the movements of the forms into one long, slow and continuous series, aimed at stimulating the health of students. He relegated fighting to a less prominent role.

This fact, and similar instances in other styles, reduces the likelihood that Tai Chi as we know it in the West today comes from Taoist mystics, swirling about in the Wu-tang peak district, oblivious to the effects their creations were to have on the western people of the late twentieth century. It may be that such Taoists were occupied with the soft type of Chi Kung (see Chapter 6), or with the Nei Chia movements.

Many people came to learn from Yang Cheng-fu and his Big Style spread far and wide. However, certain aspects of his art still remained hidden. One of his pupils and associates was a man called Yearning K. Chen, a wealthy merchant. The story goes that one day Chen asked Yang if he could borrow all the notes and writings of the family. Stuart Olson records that Yang agreed to this on condition that the notes and papers were returned to him the following day without fail. This took place in the days before photocopying machines, and even close range cameras were probably in short supply. Nevertheless, Chen took the notes and went home where he had a bevy of copyists waiting to take down the

11

Yang family papers. They must have worked all night, because Chen returned the papers the following day and shortly after this fateful night Chen disappeared.

He then published a book on Tai Chi which the Yang family claimed was a copy of their work. Chen is supposed to have denied everything. The Yang family promptly published their own book. Some people praise Chen for his initiative, saying that if he had not acted in this seemingly underhand way then the Yang family papers might never have been published, might have been lost or accidentally burned and so forth. Others say he deceived his teacher, a reprehensible act. But whatever we feel about it, the book was published, twice!

Sun Lu-tang (1860–1932) was an example of a man who first studied other martial arts and then came to Tai Chi. He was one of the chief exponents in his time of Hsing-I Ch'uan and Pa-kua Ch'uan, the other two internal martial arts of China. He studied under Hao Wei-chen, a pupil of Li I-yu. In his early years he had fits of depression and twice attempted suicide. His training in martial arts swept this tendency away and he became a famous fighter, but one who shunned attention. In his later years he blended his Tai Chi with the other two arts and founded his own recognised style, Sun Style.

Yang, Wu and Sun styles have the common Chen Style ancestor, whatever variations they may adopt. Chen Fake (1887–1957) was one of the heirs of this prestigious style. He was a seventeenth generation student and teacher. Fake regarded his art as a family heirloom and as such worthy of care and preservation. His own training schedule matched his regard. Three times a day he performed ten repetitions of any form which he was studying. In 1928 he went to Peking to teach Tai Chi. There he was challenged by three brothers who wished to test him. He disposed of the first and the other two retired before the same fate overcame them. Such is the Chinese admiration for fighting prowess that Fake was overwhelmed with requests for tuition. It was not the curative effects of his form that people wanted, but his devastating power. Until Fake went to Peking it seems that the Chen style was little known in that part of the country. But as more and more people saw Fake, and when famous actors sought his help in performing martial skills dramatically, the word spread quickly.

One must appreciate the size of China and the relatively poor communications of the day to realise that a jewel of an art could easily have lain unknown in some remote part of the land. Fake in Peking changed all that. He was recognised as a considerate and kind man, sometimes, when it came to challenges. Shen San, a prominent wrestler, confronted him one day. Fake asked the man to grip his arms and try to move him. As soon as Shen San held on to Fake's arms he knew that he had met his match. He politely withdrew. Later he commented that Fake had never told anyone about this match, this 'contest'; he said that Fake could have thrown him away like a leaf but had not done so.

A leading and innovative woman teacher of modern times is Madam Bow-Sim Mark, currently head of the Chinese Wushu Research Institute in Boston, Massachusetts in the United States. From childhood she studied the Yang and Wu styles of Tai Chi and later the Combined Form, a modern series of movements which incorporates actions from several styles. Her meticulous attention to detail and her ten hours a day training programme marked her out as a future master. She went on to study Pa-kua Ch'uan and various sword forms. She also became well known as a singer and composer of dances and was appointed the instructor of the Chinese Traditional Dancing Company. Respected and admired both in China and the United States she has been the promulgating spearhead of the new forms of Tai Chi which have emerged since the early 1950s.

This chapter shows us a number of things which are worth emphasising. One is that training in Tai Chi is a long and arduous process if a high standard is desired. Secondly, the known history of the art shows that a wide variety of movements, of differing speeds, executed with varying degrees of power were the basis of whatever is taught today. Thirdly, the influences of Taoist philosophy and religion, two separate streams, need to be much more closely examined before they can be confirmed. By this I mean that our western views on Taoism and on Tai Chi should be sifted and sorted so that when we use blanket terms we realise that we are talking nonsense.

What *was* closely connected with Tai Chi at all times was the yin-yang concept which Fung Yu-lan separates from Taoist philosophy but which I, in common with many others, regard as the first phase of that philosophy. This kind of questioning of the past raises many more questions. For instance, why have so many people written about the relationship between Taoist teachings and Tai Chi, about the I-Ching and Tai Chi, and about traditional Chinese medicine and Tai Chi? These are difficult questions to answer, but I hope that readers will find some food for thought in the following pages.

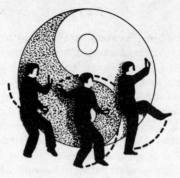

2 · THE POSTURES AND MOVEMENTS OF TAI CHI

The chequered and controversial history of Tai Chi should be borne in mind when reading the remainder of this book, especially in connection with the postures and movements. It is said that the original postures were assumed separately from one another, and that at some unknown point someone joined them together into a continuous series of movements which is generally referred to as the 'form'.

A form is found in all eastern martial arts. Some martial arts have many forms. Within the form we find all the movements and postures characteristic of the art in question. By doing the forms, students are constantly reminded of and trained in the style itself. The postures can be thought of as places on a map which one passes through, and the movements as the roads which connect the postures together. So a form is a kind of moving map. A Tai Chi teacher shows the postures to the class, corrects them and tries to ensure that they are done well. Such are the differences in physical build and temperament that no two people will take a given posture in exactly the same way. But even to an outsider, it will be plain that a posture of Single Whip for instance (see page 27) is being taken by a class of students, however much they may differ from one another.

Another strongly held belief among Tai Chi adherents is that

14

originally there were thirteen postures or movements. In the course of time, with, as we have seen, the influence of different teachers, other postures and intermediate movements were added, and variations in the positions of arms, legs, trunk and head were introduced. This tendency extended so far as to produce different styles of Tai Chi, in which the same names were given to postures which could not reasonably be called the *same*, although certain similarities often remained. An example of this is once again the Single Whip posture which has several variations, but can only be identified by the singular way in which one hand is held in a beak-like formation with the fingers and thumb joined at the tips.

Many Tai Chi enthusiasts are very partisan. Their attitude to the art is critical of other styles, and they commonly say that this or that way of doing Tai Chi is wrong. In general the more cautious students see this attitude as nonsensical, since no one knows what the original postures were like. Photographs of the famous Tai Chi master Yang Cheng-fu both as a young and an old man show differences in posture but these could be attributed to age and a change in build. His own explanation was that his posture was better when he was older. We can imagine a situation where someone who learned from Yang when he was a young man, went away for a couple of decades and then returned to him would criticise him because he was not doing the form in the same way that he had done it twenty years earlier. A fatuous criticism!

Like any other subject which is highly specialised, Tai Chi does produce in many of its followers a close attention to detail. To an outsider the exact position of a foot or hand may seem trivial. To someone who is closely involved in the art, a slight shift of the weight or the turning in or out of the foot some ten degrees makes a big difference, because an aware student experiences these small changes as a definite physical sensation. Such details then play an important part in the smooth performance of the forms and repeated wrong positions can produce injury to a joint or muscle strain, especially at the knees. Students who have been correctly taught become sensitive to details and once proficient they can usually adapt quickly to another form or style under the guidance of a competent teacher.

In my view, the taking of postures and the movements of the forms are more important, at the beginning, than any other aspect of Tai Chi. One may talk about vital energy, Chi, about the I-Ching, about the microcosmic orbit of internal energy, and other subtle subjects, but if one is unable to go through a form with a kind of hard-working yet relaxed and accurate attentiveness then such talk is simply theory or fantasy.

The most important postures are said by some teachers to be directly related to the Eight Trigrams of the I-Ching (see chapter 7). These are:

Ward Off (*P'eng*)	equated with trigram Chien	Moving in the four
Roll-back (*Lu*)	equated with trigram Kun	major compass
Press (*Chi*)	equated with trigram Kan	directions
Push (*An*)	equated with trigram Li	
Pull (*Tsai*)	equated with trigram Sun	
Split (*Lieh*)	equated with trigram Chen	Moving in the four
Elbow (*Chou*)	equated with trigram Tai	minor compass
Shoulder (*Kao*)	equated with trigram Ken	directions

This makes eight postures and to these should be added the Five Steps which are linked by some teachers and writers with the Five Elements (see chapter 7).

Advancing	related to the element metal
Retreating	related to the element wood
Looking left	related to the element water
Looking right	related to the element fire
Equilibrium	related to the element earth

The Eight Postures are sometimes called Gates, Pa-men. Wu Pu is the Chinese for Five Steps. These thirteen movement-postures are the basis for the Yang style of Tai Chi. Although the Eight Gates are theoretically connected with the eight directions of the compass, they do not follow these directions in the forms. Also, in spite of the fact that the Five Steps are sometimes related to five directions: north, south, east, west and centre, this does not have any spatial meaning in the forms either, since all movements can be done in several directions in one form.

Both Chinese and western scholars have commented on the strong Chinese tendency to conserve the past, even in the face of logical reasons for not doing so. As we shall see later, and as we saw in the history, the more prestigious the origin of an idea or theory then the more prestige it could bring to anyone associated with it. This is one of the reasons why in Chinese martial arts in general the presence of theories such as the Five Element theory are so prevalent. This is true in the field of Chinese traditional medicine also, as a later chapter will show. It has been pointed out from time to time that the Five Element theory is not an infallible one and diagnoses and treatments may have been fudged to make the theory fit.

There are few people who have the time, interest or capacity to study all the aspects of Tai Chi thoroughly and so for most of us it is a matter of accepting or rejecting or holding judgement in suspense about such theories and our own training in the forms. When one reads various articles and books about Tai Chi one cannot fail to realise that ninety-nine per cent of them are simply and uncritically repeating what was said in an earlier book, either through laziness, respect for tradition or lack of thought. Unless we have a burning desire to examine the traditions of Tai Chi then we must ourselves follow such examples or simply ignore what we do not care to investigate further.

THE EIGHT POSTURES OR GATES

1. WARD OFF (P'ENG)

In the Chen style a movement similar to Ward Off is assumed as one of the current forms begins. In it, the feet are spread wide apart as if riding a very large horse.

In the Yang style of Yang Cheng-fu we find two versions. One is exemplified by Cheng Man-ch'ing with the left hand raised in front of the chest, the right arm lowered in front of and to the side of the thigh, and the rear foot turned in about forty-five degrees. The other, seen in old photographs, shows Yang himself with the rear foot turned out at ninety degrees to the forward facing direction and the arms in a slightly different position from that of Cheng. Also, the torso is held differently. The Combined Tai Chi form, which is a synthesis produced in 1956 in China, and taught in the West by Bow-Sim Mark,

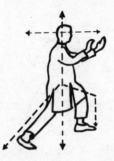

has a similar position to that held by Yang Cheng-fu.

In the version of the Wu style which travelled to Singapore, the opening movements of the form show a Ward Off posture with the trunk inclined well forward, and the hands in a different position from that of the Yang or Chen styles. Because the trigram for P'eng shows three unbroken or strong lines, yang or masculine lines (for examples of the trigrams, see page 107), then the movement itself is associated by some teachers with the supreme source of power and strength, the heavens.

When beginners first learn Ward Off and the question of what it may be used for in self defence or Push Hands occurs to them, it should be explained that in addition to its use with the palm turned in, which can denote either an attacking or defending action, it has a use with the palm turned out, an attack. Right at the moment when Ward Off is completed and the hands turn outwards to go into Roll-Back one can push with both hands at the same time. This is not apparent in learning the form because students are usually preoccupied with the transition from one movement to the other and the significance of the small hand change escapes all but the most alert. For the correct performance of Ward Off, as in all the other postures, relaxation and correct use of strength and balance should be observed. Speaking in general this has to be learned from a teacher. There are few western students who have what one could call a natural propensity for Tai Chi movement.

2. ROLL-BACK (LU)

The second movement of the Yang form, after left and right Ward Off, is done in a deep crouching stance in the Chen form. In the Yang form it is taken much higher, with again the two foot variations described for

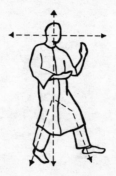

Ward Off. In the Wu style the trunk is again inclined. As the trigram for Lu consists of three broken or yin lines, this indicates that the posture or movement of Roll-Back is one of yielding, par excellence. It is the antithesis of the offensive, yang of Ward Off. At the same time in application to self defence the Roll-Back can include seizing the partner by the arm and pulling, yang, as well as the deflecting or diverting on the forearm, yin.

Within every yang some yin; within every yin some yang. This procession of defence, offence, defence, or contraction and expansion is said to reflect the natural world of seasons, waxing and waning of the moon, light and darkness, and so on. One would therefore expect the next movement to be mainly yang, and in the form this is so, with . . .

3. PRESS (CHI)

In this posture the yin and yang lines combine for the first time in the trigram with one yin, broken line on top, one yang unbroken line in the middle and a yin line at the bottom. Looked at very simply this arrangement indicates yang concealed in yin, cocooned in yin. This can be interpreted to mean that in doing Press in Push Hands the initial contact with the partner is soft, the yin line, to sense his or her balance. If this is known then the hard, yang line is used so to speak to uproot and throw off balance. Because this bright yang force is shrouded in the mist of yin, the action of Chi or Press is sometimes described as the most deceptive and dangerous.

In Chen style it is carried out in a very low stance with one leg stretched out and the other bent, the waist turning strongly to the right. In Wu style the performer presses down and then expands forward,

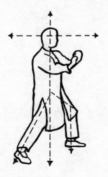

inclining the trunk with hands joined. In Yang style the left hand touches the right forearm or the heel of the hand, in all cases standing upright as a rule but one sometimes sees it with a small inclination forward of the trunk. In the simplified Twenty-Four Step Peking form the fingers of the left hand lightly rest on the pulse of the right wrist. Another variation is to press with palm against palm.

This posture is a suitable one for showing the detail and variations which were mentioned earlier. When the hands are joined in any of the ways just described it seems as though the back of the right hand and forearm will be used to uproot and throw away a partner. This is quite feasible and often Press is used in this way. However, this could be seen as a yin phase of the contact where the balance is once more sensed and then, as the hands separate to withdraw, a push could be made with both palms, facing away from the body. A different use of Press can be to use both hands, joined, to make a shock strike at the solar plexus of an opponent with the back of the right hand.

4. PUSH (AN)

In one version of the Wu style Push, it is performed with the right hand leading and the body inclined. In the Chen style it begins from the deep horse-riding position followed by bringing the feet closer and rising to a standing-up position. In both Chen and Yang styles the hands push together, though some teachers maintain that the hands should never push equally in force as this is called 'double weighting' of the hands. A similar dictum, 'no double weighting in the feet' is echoed by many teachers. This means that the weight of the body should never be evenly distributed on both feet as this make one susceptible to being

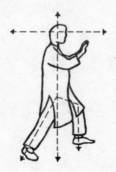

pushed off balance more easily.

In all styles the mode of pushing is subject to variations. Beginners will generally be taught to push in a straight line, subject to the teacher's preferences, and then a curving push should be introduced, something like the shape of a mounting wave. In this curving push the hands usually push down towards the waist first and then rise gradually upwards and forwards. If the action of Push is done repeatedly for training purposes then the hands will complete a kind of horizontal oval shape, dipping and rising as they go away from the body and rising and dipping as they return.

The trigram for An is one yang line on top, a yin line in the middle and a yang line at the bottom. This can imply hardness surrounding softness. For example, in making a push one might find that one is met by strong resistance, yang meets yang. Instead of increasing the power of one's own push, like two stags butting their heads together, one yields, introducing the yin as it were from the inside of the trigram. This may cause the aggressive partner to lose balance for a moment, and then with the yang from the bottom of the trigram he is made to topple over. It must be emphasised that here we are using the trigrams very ingenuously, but I see no harm in this as some of the other ways of interpreting them in connection with Tai Chi can equally be described as fanciful.

When Push is done, the body moves as a whole, as it does in all Tai Chi movements. The arms do not extend from the action of the triceps muscles alone but are powered from the legs, up the back and into the palms. The arms are simply transmitters. Push is such a committed type of movement that there is danger of losing one's balance forwards and falling through the exuberance of one's own impetuosity! Therefore care should be exercised in not letting the knee of the leading leg extend beyond the toes. A similar caution can be observed in all movements which go forward.

5. PULL (TSAI)

There are once again several variations in the performance of this action. The trigram for it is a yin line at the base with two yang lines on top. Whatever the style the movement of Tsai is a pulling one. It has been compared with the posture Needle at Sea Bottom in which the body inclines deeply forward, a rare event in Yang style, and the hands thrust down, but the posture of Lifting Hands or T'i Shou can equally be seen as a prelude to Pull. One can interpret the trigram as beginning at the base with a yin action when the first grip is taken on

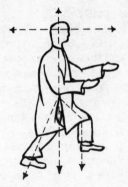

the partner's arm, and there is an immediate attempt to detect his or her state of balance and a readiness to yield. At this yin stage one is ready to release, give way or change direction, should the opportunity for yang not exist. If the conditions are right then the powerful pull with yang force incorporating the full weight of the descending body can be applied.

In the Yang Long Form, Cheng's Short Form and the Long Wu Style Form, the action of Pull can be followed by Shoulder or Elbow strokes, Kao or Chou. This means that should an initial Pull be unsuccessful and the partner draws back, one can follow up with the Elbow or Shoulder strokes to send him on his way. In the Yang and Wu forms the Needle at Sea Bottom is followed by the posture Fan Penetrates Back, which is a diverting and pushing action, also implying that an initial pull action can be followed by a combined yielding and pushing one. In the pre-arranged Push Hands form of Ta-Lu, the Dance, the posture Tsai plays an important part, and it indicates its importance as a 'fighting' movement.

Pulling may take place downwards or to the side. Whenever and however Pull is used, the whole body weight should be transmitted through the arms. This is one of the hardest lessons for beginners, who almost invariably use arm and shoulder muscle strength. One ought to remember that a body, one's own body, weighs from say 50 to 100 kg. This weight, when applied correctly, uses far less energy to produce a result than an equal weight of effort produced mainly by muscle contraction of the arms. Just imagine a huge pair of scales and in one of the pans a weight of say 55 kg. If you weigh 60 kg the only thing you have to do to lift that weight is sit in the other pan! If you tried to lift it with your arms and back it would be a completely different experience I imagine. . . . So it is with Pull. Hold the arm and – so to speak – sit down. It is 60 kg pulling down one arm.

6. SPLIT (LIEH)

Split is an action like chopping wood and it occurs many times in all forms of Tai Chi. In the form, as distinct from application to combat, whenever hands and arms descend there is an opportunity for Split. In Push Hands training it can be used to depress a partner's arm(s) and can be followed by Press, Ward Off or Push. Say that in Push Hands your partner seizes both your upper arms in an attempt to imbalance you forwards or even throw you off balance to his left. You can step out to your right, bring both arms up inside his in a curve and Split his left arm, stepping in between his legs with your left foot and Ward Off to your left. He will fly away!

Split, if timed correctly, produces an upward reaction in your partner because he will believe he is being taken down and will resist this, preparing his body for Push or Ward Off from you. Timing is probably the most important part of this action. The trigram for Split shows a strong yang line at the base and two yin lines on top. This can mean a strong, powerful beginning which upsets the partner, Split downwards, to be followed by a yielding to his reaction upwards leading to another yang action, that of Ward Off for instance. In trigram interpretation a strong yang always leads to yin just as the height of summer leads to a decline to autumn. The movement of the waist, the turning of the waist and pelvis, right or left, is important in Tai Chi and in Split followed by Ward Off, we have a decisive turn right and then left in the example given above. The two steps with the legs, right and

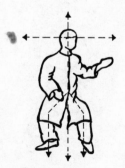

left, make this an excellent exercise in combining two of the Eight Gates.

7. ELBOW (CHOU)

Even more yang in the trigram associated with Chou once more leads to yin. Two yang lines at the bottom and one yin line on top indicate a powerful beginning concealed from view. Elbow or elbow stroke is a strong action using all the body weight, with the point of the elbow naturally in line with the solar plexus. In Cheng's form the elbow is presented to the front with the left hand 'slotted' into the crease of the right arm. In the Chen movement of Elbow Hitting the Heart the arm is bent or folded horizontally and strikes under the partner's right arm. Yang Cheng-fu's students show Elbow with the left hand held palm out alongside the striking elbow, to protect or deflect. Wu style application of the movement is similar to that of the Chen. This is not an action which lends itself to friendly Push Hands training, unless it is pulled before reaching the target or unless the partner under attack is allowed always to deflect it with his hand. It is too dangerous.

The concealment suggested by the trigram is found in the fact that Elbow is a surprise, close in attack. If your arms are being pushed it is a simple matter to let the elbow bend and move in towards the partner as he or she comes forward so that the partner 'impales' himself on the elbow point. Elbow turning can also be used to free oneself from an arm or wrist grip. If your partner grips your right wrist with his left hand you turn your elbow outwards and forwards towards his body, breaking through the 'tiger's mouth' – the space between finger and thumb, the weakest point.

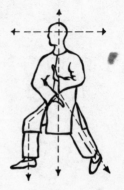

8. SHOULDER (KAO)

When the hands cannot be used, use the elbow, and when the elbow cannot be used, use the shoulder and when the shoulder cannot be used, use the torso. When the torso cannot be used, think again! Kao or Shoulder is an even closer movement than Elbow and in a sense follows naturally from it. If you attack with Elbow and your partner depresses or turns aside the attack, you simply let your body move in with Shoulder.

In Chen style this action is done in a very low horse-riding stance. In Yang style it can be done in a bow stance. In the Wu style the action begins with an almost bending-double position, ducking under the partner and rising with considerable force to send him off balance. In the Yang version the Shoulder attack is a direct blow to the front of the body, using legs, waist and back to produce a devastating shock. In Push Hands training it should be used with caution and placed on the partner's chest to give a pushing action rather than an actual blow.

Its trigram is one yang line on top of two yin lines. This arrangement can suggest the essentially hidden nature of Shoulder. When this technique is used there is no warning as there is in other movements. There is no raising of the hands, only the launching of the body by the legs. Out of this hidden initial action the powerful surprise of the shoulder hit, yang, emerges. However, it is easy to lose balance when performing Shoulder, so the yin lines can suggest an element of readiness to yield, to take care, to avoid loss of balance and to give up the attack should it seem that the partner is prepared for it. There is a temptation to lean forward too far when doing Shoulder and this invites loss of balance, so that the dictum to keep the spine erect and

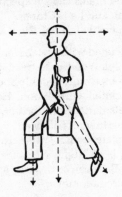

the centre of gravity low applies here. Obviously exceptions to this posture can occur.

THE FIVE STEPS

The Five Steps are so named because of the correspondence which Tai Chi theorists made between the Five Element theory of Chinese philosophy and their own art. Five Elements is not the best translation. Five Phases or Activities are preferable terms because the original Chinese characters gave more of an idea of different qualities subject to change. This is clearly very different in fundamental meaning from the western chemical one of the smallest quantity of material of a given type which cannot be further subdivided, such as we find in the Periodic Table of Elements. The names of the Five Activities, metal, wood, water, fire and earth also present western readers with a kind of mental jolt when they read them because we are used to the Greek four elements of earth, air, fire and water. Western students therefore have to leap two mental fences so to speak; that of a different number of 'elements' and variations in terminology coupled with differing meaning.

Very broadly speaking there are two camps with different views on the relevance of the Five Activities theory to Tai Chi and other Chinese cultural systems. One goes along with the theory completely, at times ignoring the fact that it clashes with the observed facts and with the more widely accepted yin-yang theory. The other sees it as a partial explanation of various phenomena and takes account of its failure to apply when the occasion arises. So any uninformed Tai Chi student would do well to remember this division. At least one Tai Chi instructor in the United States casts respectful doubt on the validity of the theory to Tai Chi, and he is Chinese. The Five Steps of Tai Chi are Advance, Retreat, Look Left, Look Right and Equilibrium.

Advance – associated with Metal. Here Metal 'conquers' or cuts through Wood, or Retreat. When the partner retreats, I advance more quickly and send him off balance.

Retreat – associated with Wood. Here Wood 'conquers' or upsets Earth, Equilibrium, by pulling and bringing the partner off balance.

Look Left – associated with Water. Here Water 'extinguishes' Fire, Look Right, when for instance a right handed Roll-Back can be upset by a left handed Push leading to a counter move.

26

Look Right – associated with Fire. Here fire 'melts' Metals, or Advance, by leading a frontal attack to the right and sending the partner off balance.

Equilibrium – associated with Earth. Here Earth 'soaks up' Water, or Look Left, which can mean that sound balance or equilibrium can absorb an attack from the left.

A little reflection, however, shows that Retreat can just as well defeat Advance in actual training, and that any of the other four steps can defeat Earth, Equilibrium if used at the right moment. Any step can be defeated by or can defeat any other step depending on circumstances. These points, however misguided they may appear to devotees of the Five Activities theory, do seem to correspond to the simple truth. In the natural world, fire is sometimes extinguished by water but at other times it boils water out of existence! At other times a kind of balance between fire and water is maintained by equal proportions of condensation and evaporation. To meet such edifying exceptions the Five Activities supporters have produced varying cycles of the Activities and cross connections which shore up their ideas. The point is that to try to force one's Tai Chi into conformity with a theory is a mistake. The Five Activities can sometimes be seen as a useful tool, and at other times a disastrous one.

ADDITIONAL POSTURES CURRENTLY IN USE

As the Yang style of Tai Chi is by far the best known and the most widely performed, and since even the modern Chinese developments in the art are largely based on Yang movements, we shall make it the subject of our discussion. Although there are other postures and movements besides the basic eight and the five steps or directions, all the additional postures contain something of the original thirteen. Anyone who trains at Tai Chi will see this eventually. Even so, the increase in the number of postures which took place from time to time under the guidance of a teacher of a new style or within an existing style has led to a growth in the exercise value of Tai Chi and to an augmented system of Push Hands and Tai Chi Combat. Even the movements which at one time were regarded as wrong or mistaken interpretations of the traditional ones have acquired respectability.

Single Whip

The most distinctive posture of Tai Chi. Traditionally done with the left hand pushing out to the front. The right hand brings the fingers

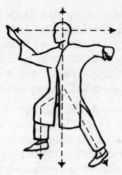

and thumb tips together with the wrist bent like the beak of a Crane. Some Tai Chi teachers hold the left hand so that the thumb is bent in giving the 'tiger's mouth' the appearance of a cobra's open jaws. It is said that Tai Chi movement comes from the actions of a crane and a snake. In Chen and Wu styles the Single Whip is performed with the legs in a horse-riding stance, the trunk facing out, away from the line of the hand actions. In Yang style most of the weight is on the front foot with the rear foot at right angles or turned in to 45 degrees. In action the use of Push and Pull can be seen. The general direction of movement in the Yang style is forward, Advance, Metal. The Crane's beak can be used to hook aside an advancing arm, whilst the other hand pushes the chest. My own first teacher told me that the outstretched right arm exerts beneficial pressure on the liver.

Lift Hands & Play Guitar

The same posture but the first is done with the right hand and leg leading and the second with the left leading. In the Wu and Yang styles the body is erect, with the heel of the leading leg touching the ground, sole raised. The hands resemble the position one would be in when holding a guitar to play it. It has the action Pull implied in it, having seized the partner's arm, and is a retreating movement, Wood.

White Crane Spreads its Wings (sometimes called Stork Cools its Wings)

A graceful and evocative posture and name. The right hand is raised high to the right like an ascending wing and the left hand lowered to the thigh like a descending one. As a child I remember hearing the impressive news that a local man had had his arm broken by the

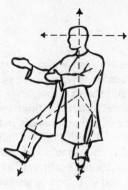

beating of a swan's wing and I stayed clear of them thereafter. White Crane is potentially both soft and hard. When a student has reached a sufficient standard of relaxation then he or she can move the arms rather like wings and produce a kind of undulating, beating effect. In the Wu style it is performed with a bend and turn of the waist and bears little resemblance to the upright, graceful movement of the Yang style. The Chen version is closest to the image of a Crane, the arms spreading out one after the other in a low, compact stance. Though conveying the idea of flying, the posture also manages to give an impression of stability, grandeur even and so one could put it into the category of Earth, Equilibrium. Yang Cheng-fu's own application of the rising hand was to parry or deflect a blow to the head, while the descending had the possibility of parrying a punch or kick to the groin. In Chinese mythology the Crane is regarded as a symbol of longevity though this does not seem to have any connection with the name of the posture. In the Yang form the posture leads into Brush Knee and Twist Step which is our next movement.

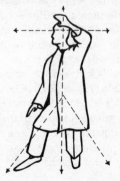

Brush Knee and Twist Step

This is a very common movement which occurs on the left and right sides. It is done in the Chen style with a high-raised knee followed by a step and in the Yang style with a low, deep step; the Wu version is performed with the characteristic inclination of the trunk forward. Like White Crane, the combined actions of the hands operate at head level and groin or thigh level. Brush Knee contains deflecting but more prominently Push. The direction is forward, Advance and so it can be equated with Metal. The modern Combined Tai Chi form has a similar high knee raise like the Chen style demonstrated by Madam Bow-Sim Mark.

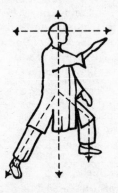

Step Forward, Deflect Downward, Intercept and Punch

A long series of connected movements employing several parts of the Thirteen Postures. In the Wu style it is done in a small space, with few steps. Chen style uses a similar series of movements done in a very low horse stance pointing to the emphasis in the style on fighting. In the Yang style, which we are using as a reference point here, the student steps forward as if pursuing a retreating opponent. Since the general direction is forward we can equate it with Advance, a Metal movement, but it also has actions of Look Left and Look Right. In relation to the Eight Gates it has the fundamental Split, Ward Off and Push within it in various guises. In spite of this fact it is a movement which, because of its elongated nature, is less close to the original thirteen. These all have a compactness, closeness to the body and simplicity which Step Forward lacks. It may be that, in common

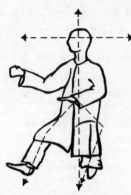

with the first thirteen, this series originally consisted of separate movements which were later strung together. Beginners find this movement more difficult than many of the other movements.

As If Closing a Door – Cross Hands

In the Yang style this is a liberating type of movement, opening the chest wide and then pulling in as though closing two sliding doors together. When the closing is completed the hands cross at the forearms. The movement and the name are very apt. In the Wu style the action is mainly on pushing rather than pulling together; maybe it is a western type of door with a hinge! The Yang version suggests a position of Equilibrium, Earth, as the arms are brought together, but as the hands reach out to left and right a Push is indicated. There are several applications of this Door movement, such as pushing aside, scooping up a leg, deflecting an arm and so forth. It is one of the more

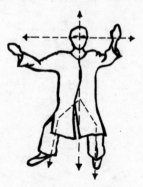

versatile actions of Tai Chi. When the arms cross there is a strong impression of balance and solidity.

Fist Under Elbow – Punch Under Elbow

In all styles the basic position of the clenched fist of one hand under the bent elbow of the other is found. The lead in to this movement, in the Yang form, is one of whirling left and right, and this gives a very good example of using the waist to move the arms. This right and left turn hints at both Fire and Water but the movement also shows a type of Roll-Back and Push action, conveying several facets of the original thirteen. The final recognised posture has strong equilibrium, too.

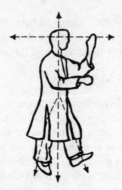

Embrace Tiger and Return to Mountain

An evocative name of a Yang style movement which has a strong Push, Look Right and then Retreat; Fire and Wood. The Return includes a

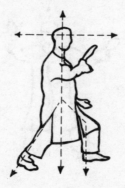

kind of Roll-Back or Pull, depending on exactly how it is performed. In all Tai Chi movements the weight is transferred from one leg to the other in rhythmic sequence and so Equilibrium, Earth, can be said to appear in all as the weight shifts. In some cases the equilibrium is centrally maintained but in others it is only passing. In the Five Activities theory, the Earth is placed at the centre through which all directions pass, so one can say that in this respect the Five Activities theory is relevant to all the postures.

Step Back to Drive Monkey Away

This movement contains a strong, retreating Wood phase or activity. In all styles where it is used, there is a Push with one hand and a Pull with the other combined with a low stance. The rear leg as one steps back takes a lot of the weight and the thigh muscles are considerably exercised, as beginners frequently testify. Tai Chi teacher Yang Jwing-ming in Boston shows this movement with a strong forward kick with the front leg, a use of the posture which is quite acceptable though not done in the form by most Yang-style students.

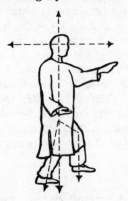

Diagonal Flying Posture

One of the most pleasing actions of the Yang form, spreading the arms wide, one high, one low and opening the chest wide after holding a ball and sinking the chest prior to performing it. Sometimes one feels with this movement that one really is going to fly. The nearest of the original thirteen to this movement would be Ward Off with the leading, rising arm, though the resemblance is not close. One could associate Advance or Look Right, even Equilibrium, with Diagonal Flying. I would choose Advance, myself, Metal. In application it can

33

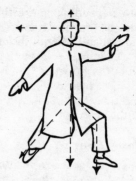

be used to strike an opponent with the top edge of the rising forearm and perhaps send him backwards over the leading leg.

Fan Penetrates Back

Was this the iron war fan or the poisoned barbed fan? Whatever the origin of this picturesquely named movement it is very enjoyable to do. The right arm rises to the side of the head and the left pushes up and forwards. One can experience the rib cage expanding and the whole torso opening as the weight is transferred on to the front leg. Both the Wu and Yang style versions have a certain similarity, with deflecting and pushing contained within them. Though the movement has a turn right or left, Fire and Water, the obviously related movement is one of Advance, Metal. Yang Cheng-fu shows the leading hand or palm hitting and the rear rising hand parrying or seizing. He describes the overall positions of the arms as like

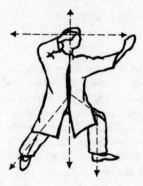

a bracket, which is a fair comparison. Beginners often place the rear hand too low down and close to the head. This would be useless in parrying a blow to the head so both for exercise and application it should be well clear of the top of the head and out to the side. If the form is done in this way then there will be plenty of reserve distance in the action when it comes to defending the head.

Wave Hands Like (In) Clouds – Cloud-Like Hands

Long, elongated or circular clouds, depending on teacher and style. If marooned on a desert island and permitted to take only one movement with them, Cloud Hands would be the choice of many Tai Chi students. I think it would be mine. Cloud Hands is a sort of self-contained series of similar movements done to the left and right sides alternately with small sideways steps. It has Fire, Water and Earth. The arms and hands describe circles across the level of the throat and lower abdomen which intersect like clouds in the sky. It would be nearer the truth to say that these circles are more like parabolas but sometimes the temptation to make them completely circular is very strong. Wu and Yang styles differ in the way Cloud Hands is done and the Chen style shows a cross-over step which is very rare in Tai Chi, though often found in other Chinese martial arts; perhaps a pointer to some of the Chen origins. Though the Chen and Wu actions have their strong points they do not have the same aesthetic satisfaction in them as the Yang action. With a little imagination one can see all of the first six actions of the Eight Gates in Cloud Hands.

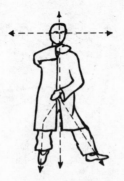

High Pat On Horse – Step Up To Examine Horse

Clearly one name was given by an animal lover and the other by a horse doctor! In direction and action this one is similar to Drive Monkey Away but has a different application. Yang Cheng-fu shows the lower hand depressing a punch and the high hand striking to the face at the same time, and the stance is higher. A retreating, Wood, motion, High Pat is sometimes seen very low in the Yang style.

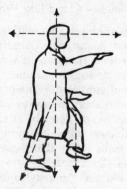

Kicks – Separate Right Foot, etc.

Several versions of kicking actions occur in Tai Chi; some of them combined with high leaps as in Chen style. In general these are not strongly emphasised in training, especially in Yang style. As a rule one can say that a leg which bears little weight in a posture is potentially a kicking leg, a leg used to block a kick or a leg used to sweep away an opponent's leg. Kicks are usually accompanied by a

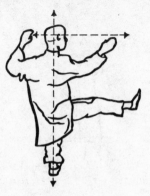

separation of the arms to the sides or diagonally. The height of kicks is usually limited to the waist in the form training, but obviously a kick can rise if necessary to a higher point. Students have to have a reasonable sense of balance to kick and in some cases must be able to swivel round on one leg, keep the balance and then kick, all in one unbroken flow. Arguments can be brought to place kicks in any of the Five Activities categories.

Strike Tiger – Tame Tiger

Of all the postures of Tai Chi this one most closely resembles movements akin to those of the Shaolin or hard-style schools. One hand is raised in a fist to protect the face and the other lowered in a fist to protect the abdomen and groin. In the Chen style it resembles a Karate movement. A similar posture is shown in Chinese and Korean temple guardians, those ancient stone statues or reliefs positioned near the temple entrances, their faces frozen in a ferocious glare to warn off intruders. It is a firm, stable posture reminding one of Equilibrium, Earth. It seems to say that no one will shift me from this position, not even a tiger! All Yang Cheng-fu's descendants seem to have used the translation given above of the name of this posture but another has been given and attributed to him. It is Hiding Tiger Reveals His Face. As the hands rise and fall the face of the tiger is seen emerging between them? Perhaps.

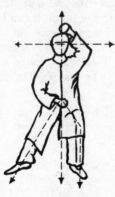

Strike with Both Fists

A movement as pleasing to the back muscles as the Cloud Hands is to the kinaesthetic sense. I remember learning this movement a long time ago and can still recall the pleasure it gave me to take the

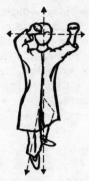

arms back and down to the sides, outwards, upwards and forwards. Both arms move together and the thumb edges of both fists strike an opponent on both temples at the same time. It is an Advance, Metal action with no apparent connection with any of the Eight Gates.

Parting Wild Horse Mane

This is a free and open movement reminiscent of Diagonal Flying but not quite as open as that. There are several variations within the Yang style but basically one hand rises, palm up, level with the throat and the other hand descends to the thigh. It can be a strike to the neck, a parry, a pull – several things at once. Its overall action is one of Advance and so Metal. Within the movements of Tai Chi there are many small movements, little turns, loops and undulations of the body which cannot properly be described in words. They need a good

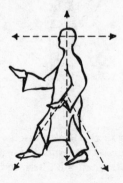

video or a teacher. Beginners cannot be expected to appreciate them all at once, and this may be why, when the modern Twenty-Four Step Peking Form was produced, all the intermediate movements which connect the postures together were taught as if they were postures in themselves. Such an approach leads to a good appreciation of the final position for each posture. For instance, in Part Wild Horse Mane the intermediate posture shows a 45 degree outward turn to the final direction and then a step forward and then a step into the final direction. This introduces Water if turning Left or Fire if turning Right followed in both cases by Advance, Metal. When we come to look at the tentative table drawn up later in this chapter we shall find Metal featuring very prominently in it.

Fair Lady Works with Shuttles – Jade Girl Works at Shuttles

Both arms are raised above shoulder level in this posture, as in Fan Penetrates Back. It is not common to find the arms raised high in Tai Chi, certainly not in the original Thirteen Postures. Critics might say that it leaves the body unprotected against kicks, that it lifts the centre of gravity and so on. But on the other hand if the head is to be protected the hands must rise and from an exercise point of view there are only a small number of ways to exercise the shoulders without doing so. So it is not a vital criticism.

Fair Lady is an advancing movement, Metal, but may be done to Left or Right, Water or Fire. It is closer to Push and Ward Off than to any of the other Eight Gates. In Yang forms it is done to the four minor compass directions with a strong turning in of the leading foot to change direction and to shift the weight. Beginners often find this intermediate movement difficult as they cannot turn in sufficiently

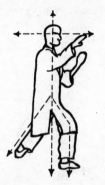

at first. These movements are reminiscent of a movement found in Pa-kua, Eight Trigram Boxing, in which the arms encircle the body, protecting it as a turning movement is made. During this same sequence of intermediate movements the balance is at greater risk than usual; so when doing them, care should be taken to keep the centre of gravity down to counteract this.

Golden Rooster Stands on One Leg

A radical departure from all that has gone before with a high posture using one leg for support and the other thigh raised to a horizontal position. The action can be used for striking an opponent in the groin with the raised knee and hitting him under the chin with the open raised palm. One can read this posture as Equilibrium, Earth, since balance is an essential part of it.

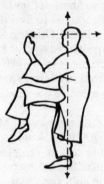

Single Whip Squatting Down – Snake Creeps Down

This posture is like the Single Whip posture except that in doing it

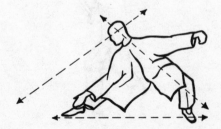

one squats down on the rear leg and shifts weight back on to the front leg. The front hand protects the groin and then moves out to attack the opponent in the groin. This is a difficult posture to do; flexibility is the order of the day, and strong legs. Approach it with caution.

White Snake Puts Out Tongue

A posture using one hand snaking out over the other and with the pointed fingers hitting a soft or vulnerable part of the body such as throat or eyes. It is an Advance and so a Metal movement.

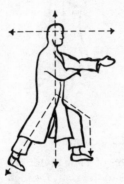

Step Up to the Seven Stars

In the Yang forms, this is a movement which usually follows Snake Creeps Down, using both fists crossed at the wrists. It can be seen as

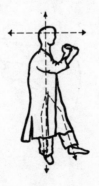

two successive punches or a blocking action using the crossed wrists. This too is an Advance or Metal action.

Step Back (Retreat) To Ride the Tiger

As it suggests, a Retreat, Wood, movement which in some ways resembles White Crane. Yang Cheng-fu shows it as a double parrying action which seems to fit it very well.

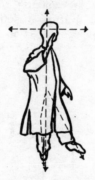

Turn Body and Sweep Lotus Leg

The only spinning action of Yang style. The weight is taken on the right foot and one spins to the right through 360 degrees, to put the left foot down, swing the right foot out and up to the left and then across the body to the right, brushing the outstretched hands with the foot. A posture not really related to any of the thirteen and so hard to place. The right leg is usually shown as a sweeping kick to

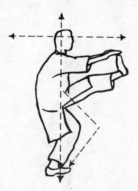

the body of the opponent. In Chen style, leaping and kicking in the air is not uncommon and it may be that Sweep Lotus is one of the vestiges of this type of action remaining in the Yang style. From a physical point of view it is hard to generate power in a kick which travels in this particular direction.

Bend the Bow and Shoot the Tiger

A posture with several variations in the Yang style alone and one which I have learned and learned again to perform in different ways. The posture looks as though you are making two punching actions, one of which is head height and the other chest height. The relationship of the hands is such that you might be holding and bending a bow with them. Yang Cheng-fu says that this action is meant to strike the opponent in the chest.

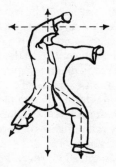

Needle at Sea Bottom

A unique movement in Tai Chi in which the body bends low to the

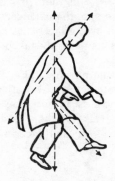

front, sometimes with the left palm and fingers touching the pulse of the right hand as in Press. It can be interpreted as a strong, pulling down action, and as it is followed in the Yang forms with the action of Fan Penetrates Back it can also be an initial upsetting movement to bring a partner off balance forward, producing a backward reaction which Fan can turn into a backward fall.

The origins of the names of the postures is a mystery. What are these tigers which keep cropping up; is the action of weaving in China like that of the Fair Lady; which Monkey is being driven away? One can see that the names can be divided into three categories. One simply describes an action, Ward Off. One describes an action from daily life, Fair Lady Works with Shuttles. One is related to Chinese culture or mythology, Embrace Tiger and Return to Mountain. I must leave it to someone else more versed in Chinese cultural history to delve into the details of this subject.

Readers may find it interesting and provocative to see an analysis of the movements of the Yang style Long Form in terms of the frequency of the Eight Gates or Postures and the Five Activities combined with other aspects of life such as the organs of the body as found in Chinese traditional medicine. This is given (on pp. 46–7). Such an analysis should be seen merely as an example of a Chinese way of looking at different phenomena and relating them; not as a definitive version. It illustrates what Chinese and western scholars have said about Chinese thought – that it looks for relationships or correspondences rather than seeking direct cause and effect.

We shall go into this question several times in later chapters. This approach describes processes rather than 'things'. It is best illustrated by referring to Chinese traditional medicine in which an overall 'picture' of a patient is produced by examination from different points of view, and then, if the picture is unbalanced, ways are found of redressing the balance, often by means of several treatments all at once. This view is of course gaining ground in western medicine and has already taken a stand in the world of physics.

Intermediate connecting movements have been left out of this analysis but they are spoken about below. It is important to note that the total number of postures depends on how they are analysed. Some may disagree with this analysis but there is a case for it as it stands. Whatever its merits or otherwise it gives a basis for speculation and comparison.

Of the Five activities we have in the table:
   81 postures corresponding to Metal – West – Lungs – Large Intestine
   25 postures corresponding to Wood – East – Liver – Gall Bladder
   24 postures corresponding to Earth – Centre – Spleen – Stomach

Then merely a sprinkling of seven mingled directions, activities and body organs from the two areas of Fire and Water. Remember that the directions in this case have nothing to do with the directions taken in the form but with the correspondences made in Tai Chi and medical theory. On the face of it, then, there are approximately three times the number of Metal associated postures as there are of Wood or Earth postures taken on their own; and a ratio of three to two if taken in combination with one another. Here we must look at the intermediate movements and the smaller movements which are not apparent until you do the forms for yourself.

It was pointed out earlier that the Centre, Equilibrium, Earth activity is constantly being passed through, and that throughout the form, the activity of Look Left and Right appears in the form repeatedly, in intermediate movements. If we count these lesser movements then the balance of activities changes. But taking the table as it stands we find a largely yang sequence of movements, partly balanced by yin movements. This seems to upset the idea of Tai Chi as a yin type of exercise, unless one brings in the question of *how* the movements are performed, and also all the smaller invisible movements. Only by doing this can we put Tai Chi into the yin camp or at least make a balance of yin and yang in it, turning on an axis of Earth, Equilibrium.

This calls into question for western Tai Chi students the widely held western view of Tai Chi as a yin form of exercise. Remember that in the section on history the Chen style, largely emphasising fighting, agility and power was the father of the modern art of Yang style. One of my own theories, which I have not yet researched fully, is that during the 1960s and 1970s when the Hippie movement was in full swing, many western young people were looking for an experience which was gentle and non-aggressive. Many of them took up Tai Chi. Intellectuals and drug inspired prophets gave endless talks and wrote articles about breezing away into a dream world of extreme *laissez-faire*. An intellectually weak grasp of Taoist philosophy and Tai Chi seems to indicate that these two aspects of Chinese culture fit that kind of bill. My own opinion is that they do not.

A further reason for the popularity of the mainly yin view of Tai Chi

YANG STYLE LONG FORM – ANALYSIS

	Times Used	Dominant Phase	Direction	Yin organ	Yang organ
Beginning	1	Earth	Centre	spleen	stomach
Ward Off	11	Metal	West	lungs	large intestine
Roll-Back	8	Wood	East	liver	gall bladder
Press	8	Metal	West	lungs	large intestine
Push	8	Metal	West	lungs	large intestine
Single Whip	11	Metal	West	lungs	large intestine
Lift Hands	5	Wood	East	liver	gall bladder
White Crane	3	Earth	Centre	spleen	stomach
Brush Knee	10	Metal	West	lungs	large intestine
Step, Deflect	5	Metal	West	lungs	large intestine
Close Door	3	Earth	Centre	kidneys/spleen/heart	bladder/stomach/small intestine
Cross Hands	1	Earth	Centre	kidneys/spleen/heart	bladder/stomach/small intestine
Embrace Tiger	2	Fire/Water	north/South	kidneys/heart	bladder/small intestine
Punch Elbow	1	Earth	Centre	spleen	stomach
Chop	4	Metal	West	lungs	large intestine
Monkey	7	Wood	East	liver	gall bladder
Diagonal	2	Metal	West	lungs	large intestine

Needle	2	Wood	East	liver	gall bladder
Fan Back	2	Metal	West	lungs	large intestine
Wave Hands	14	Earth	Centre	spleen	stomach
Pat Horse	2	Wood	East	liver	gall bladder
Kicks	10	Metal	West	lungs	large intestine
Punch Down	2	Metal	West	lungs	large intestine
Tame Tiger	2	Earth	Centre	spleen	stomach
Both Fists	1	Metal	West	lungs	large intestine
Horse Mane	3	Metal	West	lungs	large intestine
Fair Lady	4	Metal/Water/ Fire	West/North/ South	lungs/kidneys/ heart	large intestine/bladder/ small intestine
Snake Creeps	2	Metal	West	lungs	large intestine
Golden Rooster	2	Earth	Centre	spleen	stomach
White Snake	1	Metal	West	lungs	large intestine
Seven Stars	1	Metal	West	lungs	large intestine
Ride Tiger	1	Wood	East	liver	gall bladder
Bend Bow	1	Fire/Metal	South/West	heart/lungs	small intestine/ large intestine

*This table should be examined in conjunction with what is said in this chapter about intermediate, connecting movements.

47

The following is a list of the postures in the Yang style Long Form with abbreviated names in the case of very long names. For example Embrace Tiger and Return to Mountain is shortened to Embrace Tiger. If a posture is done more than once in a sequence this is shown by a multiplication sign and the number of times it occurs, for example, Monkey × 5. Read down each column beginning at the left hand side of the page.

Beginning	Kicks × 3	Monkey × 2
Ward off left	Brush Knee × 2	Diagonal Flying
Ward off right	Punch	Lift Hands
Roll-Back	Turn and Chop	White Crane
Press	Step Forward	Brush Knee
Push	Kick	Needle Sea Bottom
Single Whip	Tame Tiger × 2	Fan Penetrates Back
Lift Hands	Kick	White Snake Tongue
White Crane	Strike Both Fists	Step Forward
Brush Knee × 5	Kicks × 3	Ward Off
Play Guitar × 2	Chop	Roll-Back
Step Forward	Step Forward	Press
Closing Door	Closing Door	Push
Embrace Tiger	Embrace Tiger	Single Whip
Ward Off	Ward Off	Wave Hands Clouds × 5
Roll-Back	Roll-Back	Single Whip
Press	Press	High Pat Horse
Push	Push	Cross Hands
Single Whip	Single Whip	Kick
Punch Elbow	Part Horse Mane× 3	Brush Knee

48

Monkey × 5
Diagonal Flying
Lift Hands
White Crane
Brush Knee
Needle Sea Bottom
Fan Penetrates Back
Turn and Chop
Step Forward
Ward Off
Roll-Back
Press
Push
Single Whip
Wave Hands Clouds × 5
Single Whip
High Pat Horse

Ward Off left
Ward Off right
Roll Back
Press
Push
Single Whip
Fair Lady × 4
Ward Off Left
Ward Off Right
Roll-Back
Press
Push
Single Whip
Wave Hands Clouds × 5
Single Whip
Snake Creeps
Golden Rooster ×2

Punch
Ward Off
Roll-Back
Press
Push
Single Whip
Seven Stars
Ride Tiger
Kick
Bend Bow
Chop
Step Forward
Closing Door
Conclusion

is the beneficial effect it can have on stress. Many people associated yin with relaxation and yang with tension. This too is a mistake; one which I initially made myself. Yin can be tense and yang relaxed. We shall see later that the yin-yang theory proposes that when any condition reaches an extreme it has to change and extreme yin or yang in the human body falls into that category. A third reason for the yin view is the very great difficulty there is in combining yin and yang equally in Tai Chi performance, especially in its application to Push Hands or combat. Skill in this indicates a potential master of the art.

If this chapter has informative as well as stimulating thought about Chinese traditional philosophy and its interpretation in the West then it will have served its purpose.

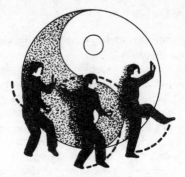

3 · PUSH HANDS AND COMBAT

When a Tai Chi student has been learning the form for some time, the teacher will introduce training in Push Hands (Tui Shou) and later on training in the combat use of the movements (San Shou). Push Hands is a very formal method of training, in which two students stand facing one another and rest their hands on one another's arms. They then push and yield alternately using a variety of methods found in the form, such as Push, Roll-Back, Press, Ward Off and so on. At first this is done without moving the feet. The aim here is to accustom them to apply force and yield to force using only the arms, torso and fixed legs. Later, Push Hands with steps is introduced and there are formal or pre-arranged movements in this phase also. One of the more elaborate training methods here is called the Dance, Ta-Lu. It is a 'dance' in the sense that students move together in certain directions, their hands always in contact in a variety of ways.

The degree of force, speed and movement used in any class will depend on the attitude of the teacher. This *can* increase as students become more proficient but some teachers prefer to keep things in a very low key. Whatever variations in action may be permitted in the class, the internal aim is the same. This is to relax the body, be sensitive to the incoming force such as a push, not to give way to aggressive emotions, and learn to make maximum use of one's own and one's partner's bodyweight. Inevitably a competitive element appears in Push Hands, but overall one tries to dissipate this by concentrating on the other factors mentioned above. One student tries to keep his balance as the other tries to make him lose it, and then the roles are reversed.

Some Tai Chi classes do not do Push Hands at all. But without it Tai Chi development is arrested. When a student does only the solo forms, it is possible to dream that balance is good, relaxation is sound and posture is correct; in short that everything is fine. When another student lays his hands on you and gives you a push, all these assumptions are tested; this is reality intruding on the dreams which may be there. Clearly there is a strong psychological factor here. For most people it is impossible to have a relaxed and yielding body accompanied by a feeling of resentment and inner refusal of what is happening. The emotional state shows up in the muscles and nerves, the postures and general demeanour, in spite of the wish for the contrary. This struggle for inner calm and non-attachment is one of the reasons why Tai Chi is called an *internal* martial art. If the inside and the outside do not correspond then the Tai Chi will not be good. The external martial arts harness aggression, fearsome expressions, muscle power and hardness. The internal need some strength too, but they also look for a calm interior, a willingness to be sensitive to the other and a desire to explore and learn. Without this the balance is lost.

Another important word which is often heard in connection with these two different approaches is 'softness'. Internal martial arts are sometimes called soft. This has led some students to interpret soft to mean floppy or weak; but this is a mistake. Soft means something which results from having the right internal–external balance. It is a kind of resilience, like the softness of rubber, yielding yet springing back into shape. Since it is contrary to our usual behaviour to be like this, training in Push Hands is a much greater test of one's Tai Chi than solo form training. It is a lifelong study, extending outside the Tai Chi class itself.

This turning of the attention inside oneself is found in Taoist, Ch'an Buddhist and Zen Buddhist teachings, among others. An excellent illustration comes from a letter written in the 17th century by Takuan, the famous abbot of a Zen monastery, Daitokuji, in Kyoto, Japan.[6] It was addressed to a swordsman, Yagyu Tajima No Kami Munenori. Writing about the inner state of a swordsman as he trains and fights, he says:

> Have no intention to counterattack him in response to his threatening move, cherish no calculating thoughts whatever. You simply perceive the opponent's move, you do not allow your mind to 'stop' with it, you move on just as you are toward the opponent and

make use of his attack to turn it on to himself . . . Kwannon Bosatsu (Avaloketisvara) is sometimes represented with one thousand arms, each holding a different instrument. If his mind 'stops' with the use, for instance, of a bow, all the other arms, nine hundred and ninety-nine in number, will be of no use whatever. It is only because of his mind not 'stopping' with the use of one arm but moving from one instrument to another that all his arms prove useful with the utmost degree of efficiency.[6]

The above illustrates clearly the principle of not fixing, of not 'freezing', of not tensing as a result of the desire to win at all costs or as a result of resentment. Constant and fluid motion is needed so that the partner in Push Hands has no solid point on which to rest his or her arms to give a strong push. Like everything else, Push Hands can turn into a habit, in the sense that a given routine with a regular partner can lull both into a happy, sleeping state in which nothing ever changes. This is why Push Hands should be varied and why it should be extended into combat type training sessions.

In this type of session there is not only pushing but gripping and pulling which brings Tai Chi nearer to the Chinese martial art of Chin-na or the art of seizing. We shall look more closely at this in chapter 5. This is not outside the traditions of Tai Chi. Yang Cheng-fu, Cheng Man-ch'ing and many other Tai Chi masters made routine use of techniques outside the purely pushing field. Even though in the West there are mixed feelings about it, in my view Tai Chi combat is necessary, if only for a small part of the training time. It is a real test of one's skill, sensitivity and attitude. In theory one should be able to elude a grip or pull without losing one's balance. Few people can but the aim is still there, drawing one on to greater efforts. There is always at least one unguarded moment when the grip of a partner is weaker, and this is the moment to escape from it.

The weight of the body itself is a factor which many students overlook. We are so accustomed to using only our muscles to accomplish something that our weight is forgotten. Even a person weighing only 50 kilograms has the possibility of moving that weight against or away from a parter. If he or she finds the right way to do this then the power of a movement can be greatly increased. Early this century the small and skinny Welsh boxer, Jimmy Wilde, used to knock down men who were very much heavier than himself. He was aptly named 'the ghost with the hammer in his hand'.

Tai Chi combat can be fast and varied, then, and the demands of moving at greater speed and coping with a variety of situations requires instant adaptation. This instant adaptation means that one must learn to be spontaneous, inventive. It has been found that if such new and spontaneous actions are remembered and examined afterwards they sometimes resemble movements found in the other two internal arts of Hsing-I and Pa-kua. It may be safe to say that spontaneity was as instrumental in the formation of new styles as the revelations of the gods in the dreams of Chang San-feng!

Instructors of modern dance who have investigated for themselves the role of the nervous system in their art have pointed out that there is a hierachy of controls in this system. Spontaneous movement comes from a different part than the place habitual action comes from, so we can express what we are trying to do in terms of moving into a different part of ourselves. Habit, desire to win at all costs, anger, pride, egoism and so forth all interrupt spontaneity and inventiveness. One sees this effect time and again in boxing matches and judo contests where the action is much easier to follow than in Push Hands training. It is often clear to a spectator that the contestant who is obviously losing the bout is continuing to employ the same ineffective and even dangerous actions which are causing him to lose but he does not adapt, does not change his tactics. His mind 'stops', to use Takuan's word, because he is gripped by fear, habit or bad advice. The man or woman who is clearly winning feels much freer, confident and inventive, letting the techniques flow without interruption and much less 'stopping' of the mind. Though this scenario is not invariably the case, it does occur often enough to give validity to the argument.

The most widely used methods of doing Push Hands in the West are those first introduced by Cheng Man-ch'ing. The methods of this man, his thoughts and the modifications which he made to the Yang style of Tai Chi have had an influence in the UK and USA far out of proportion to the influence of the rest of the existing body of teaching. This is in part due to the quality of the man but also due to the amount of promotion in the form of books and articles which he has attracted. In mainland China he is not so nearly well known nor is his form or his methods of Push Hands so highly thought of.

For reasons of his own his exposition of Push Hands stopped short, far short, of his own ability, and he seems to have left it to his pupils such as William Chen of New York to carry Push Hands further in their own ways. Some students have not carried on this development and their ability has tended to stop in the format which they first learned. This is a pity in my opinion, for it contradicts the flowing nature of Tai Chi itself.

In the martial arts, the tendency to inherit but not develop is prevalent. It is due in part to a sense of loyalty to the teacher and the past, in part to a belief that the way taught is the 'best' way, and in part to a failure to grasp the fundamental principles; principles which are the very basis of the yin-yang theory to which Tai Chi students say that their art is allied. Principles, not outward form, should guide what one does in Tai Chi, whether it is the solo form or Push Hands. At the same time this does not mean that beginners should not be given techniques and 'habits'. As Takuan wrote in this connection: '... the genuine beginner knows nothing about the ways of holding and managing the sword, much less of his concern for himself. When the opponent tries to strike him, he instinctively parries it.'[6] He has to be taught something, so that he can in the end leave it behind.

If we look at the performance of Push Hands with the steps excluded we find that most of the movements are carried out in the Bow Stance − right or left foot forward carrying most of the weight, knee bent, and the rear leg almost straight. When the weight is shifted on to the back leg, a kind of reverse of the Bow Stance, sometimes called Empty Stance, that leg carries most of the weight and the front leg is slightly bent. Bow Stance is used for the Push, Ward Off and Press advancing movements and the Empty Step for Roll-Back and retreating movements. Pushing and yielding, advancing and retreating, trace a pattern of curves, although pushing tends at the beginning to be straight. A good rule of thumb is to say that to reduce the force of a push in a straight line you lead it into a curve, and to counteract the effect of a yielding curve you reintroduce a straight line. To do this you can have no preconceived ideas since you never know in advance what will happen. Pushing in the early stages is done by resting one hand on the wrist of a partner and the other on the elbow, thus preventing a possible punch or elbow blow. Furthermore, by controlling the elbow you have a certain amount of leverage directly on the trunk of your partner through his upper arm, rather like the manoeuvrable handle on a heavy trolley. Later this hand position can be changed to pushing on the shoulder, the chest, the hips and even the knees. In general Push Hands does not include the head since it could cause injury to the cervical vertebrae in the neck. Other parts of the body are also used to push with; the elbow, the shoulder, the side of the body and even the buttocks! The last three are for very close-in work.

Push Hands without moving the feet is generally translated as Fixed Step Push Hands. In spite of the confusing translation the name has stuck, become fixed, and provided you know what it means there is no harm done. The majority of translations of Chinese Tai Chi expressions into English differ from one another as we shall see later when we make a comparison of the names of one of the weapons forms. But usually there is one word in any translation which gives a clue, such as Shuttles or Crane, to the posture or movement concerned.

The artificial restriction on leg movement in the Fixed Step Push Hands makes it imperative that students find a way to let the body give way on its own. The bending of the knees can help but also the turning of the hips and the sinking of the chest are needed. Also the free movement of the shoulder blade, scapula, can greatly assist the free movement of the arm. The next stage is to allow one or two steps backwards and forwards so that students get used to the idea of moving the feet and at the same time keeping their arms in contact with the partner's arms. The next stage can be the introduction of the Ta-lu or Dance. This varies from club to club but it is always a series of pre-arranged steps and movements involving gripping, pulling and pushing, and escaping from gripping, yielding to pulling and pushing. For example student A will push towards the South. Student B will yield to the push and step back, maybe gripping A by one arm and pull him, at the same time stepping back at right angles, to East or West. Student A yields to the pull, steps after student B and maybe attacks with Shoulder. Student B diverts the Shoulder attack and pushes and so on. The Dance shows students how to cope with changes of direction, how to adapt their footwork and keep their balance, in movement. The next stages will depend very much on the teacher. He may teach a range of other applications of Tai Chi movements or he may gradually escalate the tempo and strength of the training until the level of Tai Chi Combat is reached. This is a stage which is beyond the boundaries of this book although the interested reader could consult my own book on this subject, *Tai Chi Combat*, for further information. [Shambala, 1990]

If you look at the table on page 48 you will see that a certain number of movements occur in the Yang style Long Form much more frequently than the others. In general these movements tend to occur in Push Hands much more frequently than the others do. Ward Off, Push, Roll-Back and Press can be described as the heart of Tai Chi forms in their relationship with Push Hands. Beginners cannot at first appreciate how diversely these movements can be applied, and how slight variations in their performance, which give them a different appearance from the way they appear in the forms, do not change their intrinsic uses when applied.

Not everyone who comes to Tai Chi likes Push Hands. Some people want only the calming and relaxing effects of doing the forms. If a person's resistance to being taught Push Hands is strong then the teacher should respect it, because a student will not make much progress if he or she harbours feelings of resentment as a result of being compelled to do something which is disliked. People who have this attitude can be reasoned with. For instance it can be pointed out to them that there is something in Push Hands which is akin to the hurly-burly of daily life, where figuratively speaking we are being pushed and pulled and imbalanced by the vagaries of modern existence. This being the case, it may be possible to transfer some of the attitudes absorbed in studying Push Hands to one's encounters in life.

Few of the influences from the East which have travelled West have escaped the influences of commercialism and competition which are so rampant today. Tai Chi is no exception. Some clubs and associations now hold tournaments in Push Hands which put the aim of winning above everything else and encourage spectators so that they can collect gate money. When too strong an element of competitiveness enters, the spirit of Tai Chi leaves. It loses contact with its spiritual roots and begins to work in the entirely opposite direction. The defeat of an opponent becomes the primary concern and all ideas of understanding oneself are in general forgotten. This is what happened to Judo a long time ago. It is up to those students who want to preserve the spirit of the art to ignore these carnivals.

My own contact with Push Hands was at first sporadic. It seemed to me to be at odds with the fundamentals of Tai Chi which I saw as primarily yin, yielding. Over the years my attitude changed. I began to see it as a discipline of non-aggression and a means of using strong action without the emotional intent to injure. When I began to teach, it brought me a great deal of satisfaction to see men and women, some of them big and strong, learn to check the desire to win or not to lose in favour of learning something about the interplay of yin and yang. This was accompanied by an increasing sensitivity and bonhomie in the classes. To see the timorous gain in confidence over a long period of time was another plus for me as a teacher. Although I am a teacher in that I pass on what I can to others, my approach has continued to be that of a student at the same time. If a member of the class discovered a new technique during Push Hands then we all studied it. There seems to be no limit to discovery in Tai Chi.

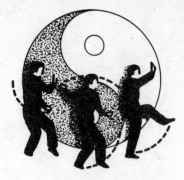

4 · TAI CHI WEAPONS

In the Chinese martial arts tradition, skill with a weapon has always been placed on a higher level than skill with the empty hand. This is partly because more skill *is* required, and partly because in the past a nobleman or gentleman would not as a rule 'stoop' to bare first fighting. Bodyguards were employed to deal with such distasteful things. Exceptions to this disdain can be found but they are definitely exceptions. Today this attitude has changed in the sense that there is no longer a class distinction invading the question. In the mainland Chinese Wushu (martial arts) training syllabus the students are introduced to empty hand forms first and to weapons later; purely on a basis of the degree of difficulty. Many of the hand positions, stances and body movements of unarmed forms are used in the weapons forms and a beginner is better served by being taught the former first. Once the body is trained then, when the weapons are taken up, a student can concentrate his attention on the intricacies of the sword, spear or pole techniques without having to think about the basic factors.

Not all teachers teach the same weapons in Tai Chi. But a common selection from the vast array of Wushu arms is the Jen, a classical double-edged straight sword; the Dao, a single-edged curved sword resembling what we in the West would call a scimitar; the Ch'iang, spear; and sometimes a long type of halberd.

It is worth reminding readers here that the translations of Chinese nouns into English is today a very haphazard affair in the martial arts literature. For instance the word for Jen can also be found spelled

Chien. Unless you are very much alive to pronunciation this can cause much confusion. The letters 'ch' are frequently found in Chinese nouns. When they are followed by an apostrophe, as in Ch'uan, fist way, the 'ch' is pronounced softly as in 'church'; when not followed by an apostrophe, as in Chien, the 'ch' is pronounced like the 'j' in 'job'. So as a rule of thumb an apostrophe following a consonant can be taken as a signal that one should pronounce softly and the absence of an apostrophe a signal that pronunciation should be hard.

The Tai Chi sword, Tai Chi Chien (Jen) varies in length and ideally should suit the height and weight of the user. The swords available today include antique swords, modern swords of spring steel, alloy swords, swords composed of two laminated metal strips and wooden swords. Sometimes you may see a sword with a tassel attached to the end of the handle. These are mainly used in sword dancing and public demonstrations as they add to the spectacle. For training purposes it is better to remove the tassel as it can get in the way and wrap itself about the wrist. Another explanation for the use of the tassel is that it balances the sword in the hands of a sensitive performer, but opponents of tassels say that it should not be used at all since in combat it could be seized by an enemy to wrest the weapon from the user's grasp, or at least give an enemy some temporary control which could be fatal.

If you cut a transverse section through a sword blade you have a shape like a flattened diamond of the kind seen on playing cards. The blade comes to a point at the end with a rapid taper, the two edges being parallel until the taper begins. The guard, which is ideally never much wider than the fist formed around the handle, turns down towards the blade and not back towards the hand as in many western bladed weapons. If a bladed weapon is shorter than the forearm of a man it is usually classed as a dagger. The space formed by the hand around the handle of the sword is called the Tiger's Mouth.

A right-handed student holds the sword mainly in that hand but at the beginning of most sword forms it is held by the left hand using a reverse grip. This means that the flat of the blade runs up along the left arm pointing towards and beyond the armpit and shoulder. After a few movements of the form, the left hand places the handle in the open right palm. Then the left hand takes on a particular shape. This consists of the index finger and middle finger held straight in line with the palm and the remaining two fingers being folded across the palm with the thumb pressed down on top of them. This hand formation is known as the sword charm, the sword amulet or the helper of the secret sword. In sword form theory this sword charm is supposed to conduct vital energy, Chi, into the right sword arm at the point of the pulse, the

TRANSLATIONS OF SWORD FORM MOVEMENTS

Dr Tseng Ju-pai

Commencement
Three haloes round the moon

Big dipper
Swallow gives a delicate touch on the water
Right and left intercept and sweep
Little dipper
Swallow entering the nest
An agile cat catching a mouse
Phoenix raising head
A wasp entering a cave
Phoenix spreading wings

Little dipper

Waiting for fish
Push aside grasses for finding the snake

Birds flying to forest for roost
Black dragon wagging tail
Green dragon appears on the water surface
The wind rolling up the lotus leaf
A lion shaking head

Wild horse leaping the stream
Turn round to rein in horse
A compass

Yearning K. Chen

Beginning posture/step forward and unite/the sword
Immortal guiding the road (to) triple brace
    lets embracing the moon.
Major star of the dipper
The swallow searches for water
Obstruct and sweep
Minor star of the dipper
Wasp entering the hive
The spirit of the cat catches the rat
The dragonfly sipping water
The swallow entering the nest
Phoenix spreading both wings
Whirlwind to the right
Minor star of the dipper
Whirlwind to the left
Fishing posture
Stir up the grass and search for the snake
Embrace the moon
Send the bird up into the trees

Black dragon wagging its tail
The wind rolls up the lotus petals
The lion shaking his head
The tiger embraces its head
The wild horse leaps over the mountain stream
Turn the body over to stop the horse
The compass

Facing wind to dust
Drifting with the current
Meteoroid pursuing the moon
Divine horse gallops in the sky
Raise up the curtain
Sword wheeling left and right
Swallow holding clay in the mouth
Fabulous bird spreading wings
Salvage the moon from the sea bottom
Carry the moon in the bosom
Na-cha sounding the sea (Na-cha: legendary supernatural being)
Rhino looking at the moon
Shoot the wild goose
Green dragon shows its claw
Phoenix spreading wings
Intercept left and right
Shoot the wild goose
White monkey offering fruits
Blossoms fall left and right
A damsel throws the shuttle
White tiger cocks the tail
The carp bounds on the dragon's gate
Black dragon entangles the pillar
The fairy shows the road
An incense offered to heaven
A whirlwind blows the flowering plum
Offer an ivory tablet with both hands
Take the sword to normal – Denouement

Greeting the wind and wiping away the dust
Drift with the current
The meteor pursues the moon
The skylark flying over the waterfall
Raise the bamboo curtain
The cartwheel sword, left and right
The swallow holds mud in its mouth
The great roc spreading its wings
Dragging the moon from the bottom of the sea
Embrace the moon
Yak-sha searches the sea

Rhinocerous gazing at the moon
Shoot the wild goose
The blue dragon stretches out its claws
Phoenix spreading both wings
Cross and obstruct left and right
Shoot the wild goose posture
The white ape offering fruit
Falling flowers posture
Fair lady weaving at shuttles
White tiger twists its tail
A carp leaping over the dragon gate
The black dragon twisting the pillar
The immortal guiding the way

The wind sweeps away the plum blossoms
Holding up the ivory tablet
Embrace the sword and return to the original posture.

wrist, during many of the movements of the form. Chi is said to flow from the two pointing fingers and into the acupuncture channels. The pressure of the sword charm can also help in the technique in which the sword tip is moved in a circle. The tips of the pointing fingers press down on the end of the sword handle to assist this action. Furthermore, since the Tai Chi sword is wielded mainly by one arm and therefore puts more of a demand on the muscles of the right side of the trunk, the sword charm position and its movement in harmony with the sword arm helps to activate and use the left side of the body, giving a certain degree of energy balance.

The movement of the body during a sword form should be lithe, fluid and lively. This applies when the form in question is quick. When the form is slow, calm and measured, as in some versions of the Yang style sword form which follow the same pace as the Long Form, students are taught to make their movements correspond as much as possible to the feeling of that empty hand form. The Tai Chi writer Yearning K. Chen states that in the Yang style there are thirteen sword actions.[7] Others give sixteen or twenty but this discrepancy comes about by the way in which the actions are divided up. For instance a parry and a chop can be combined into one action in one style and treated as two separate actions in another. Also, since the classical sword is used not only by Tai Chi students but by other martial artists from different hard-style schools there has no doubt been an exchange of techniques between all of them.

The lithe and fluid use of the sword is very difficult to achieve and there are few westerners who can reproduce the movements of the Chinese experts. In a rare film of T.T. Liang performing the Tai Chi sword form of the Yang style, he makes the whole exercise look so easy and so relaxed that he looks as if he were playing. It is only when one picks up a sword oneself and tries to use it that the skill of this Tai Chi master is realised. Similar remarks could be made about Madam Bow-Sim Mark who is known the world over for her electrifying sword work. In her one sees the acrobatic influence of modern Wushu training while in master Liang one perceives a different, earlier influence coming from years of dedicated study of the solo form.

A key point in sword use is a strong and flexible wrist and elbow. The sense of balance needs to be more highly developed than in the empty hand form since the momentum of the blade as it sweeps and cuts tends to pull the body out of alignment.

Below are some names given by Yearning K. Chen[7] to the thirteen actions in the Thirteen Posture Sword Form:
Once again one should bear in mind that the English translations of these terms may vary from book to book and teacher to teacher. Perhaps everyone is intrigued and sometimes charmed by the names of the movements of the forms and the names of the sword techniques. Listed on pp. 60–61 are the translations of two writers of the names of the movements of the Yang family sword form, for the reader's interest and comparison. Sometimes an intermediate movement is listed by one author and not by the other.

Ch'ou	– lashing	Peng	– snapping
T'ai	– striking	Chiao	– stirring
T'i	– raising	Ya	– pressing
Ke	– blocking	Pi	– splitting
Chi	– piercing	Chieh	– intercepting
Tz'u	– stabbing	Hsi	– clearing
Tien	– pointing		

For one thing there are some understandable misunderstandings! The movement given as 'black dragon entangles the pillar' and the 'black dragon twisting the pillar' seems to have been the victim of unclear translation. It is not clear whether the dragon's body is twisted around the pillar or by its action is twisting the pillar around. The movement in the form consists of turning the sword in different directions as if encircling a pillar, that is, the opponent, so perhaps the first interpretation was intended. This is a minor point and is not meant as a criticism of either writer. In a way the unclear translation adds to the charm of the names. Some of the names are graphically accurate; that is to say the posture explains its own name. For instance the posture called The Compass is taken with the feet close together, both hands holding the sword at arms' length, horizontally, with the sword also horizontal; just like a compass needle pointing to magnetic north. Whirling to the Left is a whirling movement and Fishing posture is like a fisherman holding a rod in his right hand outstretched in front of him while the left is held outstretched behind him to keep his balance. The dragons, meteoroids and Na-Cha (Yak-sha) plainly refer to the mythology of China and had a particular aptness for the original givers of the posture names. Yearning K. Chen states: 'The venerable Yang family were the first Tai Chi authors to hand down the names of these swords skills'. Chen also lists the long staff as a Tai Chi weapon.

STANCES AND ACTIONS

The Yang family sword form requires the expenditure of much more energy than the empty hand form. This is not just because a student is holding a weapon but because there is much more activity in it. One cannot help thinking that this is because the sword form is closer to the original Chen style with its greater emphasis on varied movement and changes in tempo. Video tapes of Chen style from Taiwan and mainland China confirm this theory.

The chief stance of the form is the Bow Stance, sometimes called the archery stance, taken rather wide and deep, weight on the front leg as in the empty hand form. Some instructors, mainly from the Shaolin or hard style schools of Kung fu, say that in this stance the weight is evenly distributed on both legs. The only way to manage this is for the bent front leg to push back as it were against the pelvis and transfer force back on to the rear leg. This is not the way it is done in Tai Chi. Another stance which is used in the sword form is the tip stance or T-stance with the weight on the rear leg and the front leg resting on the ball of the foot or toes, heel slightly raised. The stance which can be seen in a sense as the reverse of the Bow Stance is the Waist Drawn Back stance or Empty Stance, again with weight on the rear leg but with the whole of the sole of the front foot touching the ground. The Horse Riding Stance, like a person sitting on a large horse, has the feet spread wide apart, more or less parallel, and this stance occurs a few times in the sword form. The stance with one leg raised, thigh more or less parallel with the floor, does not seem to have been given a name by either of the above writers but it could safely be called a Crane Stance; it also appears several times in the sword form. The remaining noteworthy stance is assumed by bending the rear leg deeply, almost a squat, and the front leg sliding forward. It is similar to the stance for Snake Creeps Down or Single Whip Squatting Down in the empty hand form. The stance is sometimes called the Sliding Stance.

Returning to the question of the names of the postures, it is very striking that the imagery which they conjure up is often very peaceful, even domestic; Fair Lady Working at Shuttles, for example. In this respect they contrast markedly with the purpose of the movements they describe, for after all the sword and fist are used to injure or kill. Why use imagery of peaceful, constructive activities for activities associated with war and violence? I have no definite answer to this and can only suggest two lines of thought. One of these is the aptness of the comparison between the activity and the sword action in question.

The other is the widespread tendency to disguise and be secretive about almost everything in martial arts lore. I have never found any explanation which is conclusive.

The Dao or scimitar or Big Knife as it is sometimes called is about one metre long; curved, sharp along one edge and the blunt edge or back some twelve millimetres thick. Dr. Tseng Ju-pai records that blades should not be swung so that the cutting edge cross the fontanel; the place on the top of the skull where the bones meet and which is so soft and delicate in a new born baby. This point, approximately in the middle of the head, is traditionally thought of as the point through which his spiritual energy connects a man with heaven and it would be a profane act to sever it with a sword. However, if the blunt edge of the Dao is swung back over this point, this is acceptable since it does not have the power to cut through spiritual energy. It is believed that the Dao originated in the Bronze Age. Stories are told of how the Dao was used during the Chinese war with the Japanese in hand to hand combat. It is said that it was very effective, especially in the hands of trained guerilla fighters. Among the tales of unusual swords of this type is one that in ancient times a warrior, Kuan Kung, had a Dao weighing some sixty kilograms. The form for the Yang family Dao uses thirteen actions. Yearning K. Chen names them thus:

K'an	– chop	Lu	– claw
To	– cut	Pi	– split
Ch'an	– slice	Ch'an	– bind
Chieh	– intercept	Shan	– fan
Kua	– parry	Lan	– obstruct
Liao	– stir up	Hua	– slip upwards
Cha	– pierce		

The names of the actions are different from those of the Jen form. Dr Tseng Ju-pai writes: 'As they (the people who handed down the names) were mostly illiterate and spoke a dialect, the right names of the postures are very difficult to put down in (English) writing. Now we have to give them temporary names for easy memorising.[8] Indeed the names given in some manuals of instruction are purely descriptive of the action; for instance, slash right, left and upward and advance to stab upward. Many of the techniques of the Dao involve a slashing movement. The nature of the Dao's use is very fierce, like a tiger, and the use of the weapon in the Yang family form does not show the weapon off to its best advantage. Madam Bow-Sim Mark demonstrates the use of the Dao as found in the modern Wushu training syllabus and one can see its great dynamic potential. Speaking in general one can say that greater physical fitness and agility is needed to use the Dao well than to wield the Jen well. However, this is offset by the elegance of the Jen form. Very few Tai Chi students know or study the Dao form. This may be because they feel that it is not in harmony with their feeling for Tai Chi or that not many teachers know it either. It takes many years to master a weapon and the idea of spending seven years on the sword and seven years on the Dao is very daunting.

The writer Robert W. Smith noted that 'The British in the mid-nineteenth century acknowledge that the Chinese spear was far superior to their bayonets.' The spear, Ch'iang, varies in length from about two to three metres. The haft, whatever wood is used, should be pliable and resilient for Tai Chi. A rigid type of wood is not suitable. The head of the spear is roughly diamond shape with a taper to a point. Almost invariably around the place where the head is fixed to the shaft a bundle of tassels is tied. Frequently, horse mane or tail hair is used and dyed red. When a student shakes the spear during training the vibration of the hair indicates something about the quality of his chi and his muscular strength. It is also said that the hair absorbs blood, and this may explain the use of red dye to signify the colour which it would become in battle.

If the use of the Dao is comparatively rare, then use of the spear is rarer still. Dr Tseng Ju-pai was taught two uses of the spear by Yang Cheng-fu. The first he called unilateral drill and the second bilateral drill. The unilateral drill consisted mainly of shaking the spear. This action of shaking is connected with the pliability of the wood used for the haft of the spear. When the weapon is shaken by an expert you can see the energy travelling down the vibrating wood to the point. If the wood were dense and rigid and so to speak insensitive to the movement it would not convey this vibration and the user would not be able to transmit his energy to the point in quite the same way. Tai Chi shaking of the spear would be impossible.

In the bilateral drill there are thirteen actions of attack and defence grouped in four categories. These are: tenacity, rebound, tenacity and rebound combined, and entanglement. Tenacity echoes the idea of Push Hands training where one tries to remain in contact with one's partner; sticking. Rebound contains the notion of using the opponent's energy to move one's own weapon. Tenacity and rebound studies the combination of the first two. Entanglement involves wrapping one's own spear around the spear of the partner, although this notion cannot be carried too far and usually means advancing with a circling action with the two spears in contact. The spear point in this action of Entanglement moves in a spiral or series of circles, reminiscent of the basic techniques of the western fencing foil. Sometimes the spear, held in the right hand, is thrust through the lightly clenched palm of the left hand between the first finger and the thumb. The movement is comparable with sliding a snooker cue over the hand.

In all Tai Chi weapons there is an aspect referred to above as 'sticking'. A student is taught to try to remain in contact with his partner's spear, and then the 'follow'; another common expression. Wherever he goes I follow. This is a very difficult art and one reads of amazing feats of sticking where a master cannot be dislodged once he has stuck to an opponent. The basic idea is that once the weapons come into contact then the Tai Chi student follows every action of his partner, sensing or anticipating everything that happens, appreciating the fluctuations of yin and yang and moving with the partner as if they were fused together. In a less elaborate way this is found in western fencing where a parry is made and the defender, keeping his blade in contact with that of his opponent, slides in with a thrust. As long as you can stick to your partner, you have some control over him, or, at least the sensation as well as the vision of what he is doing. In martial arts contests, when they are not artificially slowed down, action is very, very fast indeed. Like a striking snake! Visual perception is almost too slow to keep track of what is happening and the sensation of the opponent's body, fed in through the hands, is an invaluable aid.

When a Rebound technique is used, the shaking action is combined with a type of blocking movement which can turn the opponent's weapon aside with some force and present an opening for attack. Then the sticking techniques have served their purpose. Another method of pre-arranged training with the spear is for both students to rest their spears against one another about half a metre from the head and turn them in a circle, keeping contact. As the circling continues, one of the students will judge that there is an opening, a weakness in the other's concentration, and will thrust forward.

In the United States, Stuart Olave Olson, under the guidance of his teacher T'ung-Tsai Liang, began a revival of interest in the Tai Chi Spear, producing a book, *Wind Sweeps Away the Plum Blossoms* and companion video tape in 1985. He traces the origin of Tai Chi spear techniques to the famous Shaolin Temple monks, through the Chen family and thence to the Yang family. It is said that of all weapons the spear is the best for developing internal energy. The Shaolin Temple spear techniques were called Plum Blossom, as a group, and their names have the characteristic poetic imagery.

Olson translates them as:

Yaksha Searches the Sea
All the Barbarians Paying
  their Respects
The Compass
Ambush from the Ten
  Directions
The Blue Dragon Offering its
  Claws
Intercepting to the Side
Overturning the Iron Staff
Bestriding the Sword
Spreading Brocades on the
  Ground
Facing Heaven
An Iron Ox Ploughing
  the Soil

Dripping Water
Riding a Dragon
A White Ape Dragging a Sword
Playing the Guitar
The Vigilant Cat Seizes the Rat
Crushing an Egg with Mount T'ai
A Beautiful Woman Threading
  a Needle
Blue Dragon Wagging his Tail
Breaking into the Hung Men (Gate)
A Crouching Tiger
The Sparrow Hawk Seizes a
  Quail
Chaing T'ai Kung Goes Fishing

Several of the names are the same as or close to the names used for the Jen, double edged sword, and the empty hand forms. The image of dragons, a word not appearing in the Yang family empty hand forms, does occur in the Chen family forms.

A final word about weapons training is to say that they need a lot of space. For empty hand forms a relatively small area can be used for training but when wielding a sword or scimitar the space increases four or five times that amount. In addition to the space needed by each student there must be a gap of a metre or two to allow for safety margins. This may be another minor factor in the small number of people practising Tai Chi weapons today.

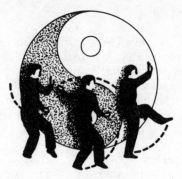

5 · TAI CHI AND ALLIED MARTIAL ARTS

Whenever martial arts students and teachers get together, whatever their style or art, you do not have to be a genius to guess their chief topic of conversation. Stories and gossip about martial arts are handed around, endless comparisons between techniques are made, arguments about the past rage in a friendly way, and occasionally someone will rise to his feet and demonstrate a point. In short, the *bonhomie* of 'insiders' the world over permeates the group. In such surroundings you always hear about something which you did not know about before; about different arts, teachers and events. This was the same in the past, and may partly explain why students who have been devoted to one style for a long time sometimes leave it and go to learn something else. Martial arts get into your blood, and once you have trained seriously for a while you never want to give them up completely. If you find another challenging and interesting outlet for this restlessness, and searching, you should go and find out about it.

A modern, documented example of this was Kenichi Sawai, a Japanese man born in 1903. At the age of twenty-two he was already a 5th Dan Black Belt in Judo, a 4th Dan in Kendo and a 4th Dan in Iaido, the art of drawing and using a real sword. With this background he went to China when he was twenty-eight, on business, and heard about a martial artist called Wang Hsiang-ch'i. Wang was a famous Hsing-I teacher of the Honan school. The other famous school at that time was the Shansi-Hopei school. When Wang was proficient in Hsing-I he changed the name of his art to I-Ch'uan (Mind Boxing). Whichever name is used, the general implication of the Chinese words is that of body and mind moving in harmony, which is of course true of Tai Chi and other martial arts. The differences in all these arts lies in the emphasis.

After a short period of 'Knocking on the door', Kenichi Sawai managed to arrange a meeting with Wang, and the inevitable test of skills ensued. Sawai wrote: 'When I had my first opportunity to try myself in a match with Wang, I gripped his right hand and tried to use a technique. But I at once found myself being hurled through the air . . . Next I tried grappling. I gripped his left hand and his right lapel and tried the techniques I knew, thinking that, if the first attacks failed, I would be able to move into a grappling technique (fighting on the floor) when we fell. But the moment we came together, Wang instantaneously gained complete control of my hand and thrust it out and away from himself.'[9] Kenichi Sawai was still not deterred and requested a contest with sticks, to stand in place of swords. The Japanese sword expert could not touch Wang. However, Wang was good enough to accept Sawai as a pupil.

Within the teaching of Hsing-I or I-Chu'uan of Wang Hsiang-ch'i was a branch known as Ta-ch'eng-ch'uan. Sawai studied this and when he was competent in the art, Wang gave him permission to start teaching it in Japan and to give it a Japanese name which would be comprehensible in that language. He chose the name Tai-ki-ken, which is the Japanese rendering of Tai Chi Ch'uan. It must be said that the Tai-ki-ken which is shown by students of Kenichi Sawai does not resemble Tai Chi very much, but we will go into the technical side later. The foundation training for Wang's Hsing-I was standing meditation. Kenichi Sawai called it Zen standing meditation, even when writing about it in connection with Wang, but as the latter was Chinese it must originally have been Ch'an Buddhist or Taoist meditation of some kind. This meditation method in a standing position is said to arouse very active modes of Chi, vital energy, and give students a kind of springing, animal power of movement which is hard to stop.

When he began standing meditation, Sawai suffered very much physically, in spite of all his previous hard martial arts training; perhaps because of it! His sober reflections as he studied and stood for an hour at a time in one posture were that 'when a person begins . . .

he will experience pain in his hands, his feet or his hips. When this happens, all of his thoughts concentrate in the parts of the body that hurts, and he is unable to think of anything else.'[9] Eventually, after eleven and a half years of this standing exercise, Kenichi Sawai came to a new understanding of the art. But he stated in his writings that not only martial artists do this type of exercise. It is common in several religious Ways. One of the results of this practice is to clear the mind of thoughts, but not necessarily as a consequence of pain. When standing still the aim is to achieve relaxation.

There are five basic techniques of Hsing-I: splitting, crushing, drilling, pounding and crossing. This is the terminology given by Robert W. Smith, but other English words are sometimes used such as: smashing, threading, snapping, rushing and poking. In addition to these five techniques there are twelve methods of moving based on the actions of animals: dragon, tiger, horse, monkey, cock, hawk, iguana, snake, eagle, bear, swallow and ostrich. A technical characteristic of Tai-ki-ken is the low, crouching stance adopted for many of the movements, reminiscent of the tiger movements, but also reminding us of Tai Chi. Today, many exponents of Tai Chi stand high; that is, with only a slight knee bend and tucking in of the joints at the groin. But if you look at old photographs of Yang Cheng-fu and Chen Wei-ming you will see that they are low, denoting power in the legs, and the waist.

When I had been doing Tai Chi for a number of years I met a teacher who had been training with one of the Yang family descendants at the university in Hong Kong. He brought my stance down very low, and I appreciated the leg strength and hip or waist power needed to perform the movements in the older way. In Tai Chi Combat, a method of driving down an opponent's arms was discovered in 1989 which is very similar to the Hsing-I action of Splitting. Some of the techniques of Tai-ki-ken are very similar to this movement, combining their low, tiger-like stance with a splitting action, 'rising and falling as if chopping with an axe'.[9] Where Tai-ki-ken and Tai Chi differ is very much in the fact that there is not the same softness in the action, and also Tai-ki-ken is completely geared for fighting. Kenichi Sawai furthered his inherited art and in so doing he indicated the infinite possibilities of combination and permutation within the martial arts as a whole.

Sun Lu-t'ang, (see Chapter 1) was a student and teacher of three arts: Tai Chi, Hsing-I and Pa-kua. He was renowned in his own lifetime and his Chi power marked him out as an unusual person by any standards. Some of his early training emphasises a point which cannot be emphasised enough to Tai Chi students. This is that although Tai Chi is soft, an internal style, the softness requires very hard training to acquire. One of Sun's teachers, when he was learning Hsing-I, was Kuo Yun-shen. Kuo would mount a horse, make Sun hold on to the horse's tail, and ride for long distances with his pupil tagging on behind. Sun's skill increased as he was trained but one day he met his match. He heard a man coming up behind him to attack, and tried to seize the man. The assailant avoided his move and try as he might, Sun could not grip him. The stranger turned out to be a Taoist. He taught Sun how to cultivate his Chi even further and gave him dietary advice which included the suggestion that he should not eat meat. Sun's powers also extended to healing, horse riding, fighting with a staff, and archery. 'From a distance of a hundred paces,' writes Robert W. Smith, 'he could shoot a coin off of an egg held by a student.'

These two examples of martial artists with a mixed background bring into focus the question of the purity of an art such as Tai Chi. Wherever we look we cannot find the 'pure' style or stylist. Whoever we examine we find that either he, or she, or their teaching itself has been influenced by another martial art entirely, or by another style of Tai Chi which has disappeared or which still exists alongside them. One hears time and again in Tai Chi circles, from people who do not think or do not know, that they are doing the original pure Yang or Chen or Wu style. The truth is that there is no such animal. Everyone is doing a variation on something else. Sometimes examples of changes can come about from ludicrous causes, and I quote one from my own experiences.

Occasionally I train and teach in my back garden. One of the forms I do requires a little more space than the width of the garden can allow. When I reach the garden fence I am doing Ward Off, Roll-Back, Press and Push. To do this I have to raise my arms higher than I should do so that I can clear the top of the fence. One evening a pupil was watching me and began to imitate this incorrect raising of the arms. If he had gone away without having the reason for my action pointed out to him, and had never come back again, a new variation in the form would have been created!

Yang style Tai Chi is the most popular outside Asia. It features very few clenched fist techniques. The chief formation of the hand found in the style is the open palm. This is also the chief hand formation in another internal art, Pa-kua Chang or Eight Trigram Boxing. A striking feature of this style is that students learn to 'walk the circle'. That is, the central method of training is to walk continuously in a circle, and then, following specific foot movements, to turn and retrace the same circle in the opposite direction. The open palms are held in such a way as to protect the head and trunk and as the change in direction is made the hands twine around the body and back into their original position. This action of the hands is called Palm Changing, of which there are several variations of increasing complexity.

In Tai Chi traditional training the use of the waist to effect turns, evasions and attacks is emphasised but in Pa-kua it is stressed even more. From a theoretical point of view the Eight Trigrams (see page 107), which were the basis of the sixty-four Hexagrams of the I-Ching, are mentally located at regular intervals around the circle which the Pa-kua student walks. Each Trigram is placed at a particular point on the eight compass directions and has its own special meaning and qualities associated with it. The idea is that the student trains and is mindful of these eight places as he walks the circle. Without making too much of an argument about it, one can see similarities between this exercise and shamanist or magical rites. If we take the I-Ching's description of the Eight Trigrams we have the attributes of Strong, Yielding, Inciting Movement, Dangerous, Resting, Penetrating, Light-giving, Joyful, and corresponding images of Heaven, Earth, Thunder, Water, Mountain, Wind, Fire, Lake. Picture the Pa-kua student as he moves round the circle, keeping his body relaxed and vertical, and imagining these different qualities as he passes their corresponding points. His leading hand is directed to the centre of the circle and his gaze follows his hand, to a place from which all this emanates. We have here all the hallmarks of some kind of ritual which is far removed from ideas of combat.

Since the Eight Trigrams were originally thought of as representations of all that happens in the heaven and on earth, perhaps students of Pa-kua are meant to be immersing themselves in this representation as they move. In the main, this kind of mental process is not followed by Pa-kua enthusiasts in the West.

Though the origin of Pa-kua is not known it is traditionally placed in the Ch'ing dynasty. Its documented history begins in the late eighteenth century with the appearance of a certain Wang Hsiang, from whom it was handed down to the present day. The techniques of the art includes striking, seizing, tripping and throwing. It is known as a very fierce and powerful style. We in the West are not familiar with the use of the palm (heel) as a striking surface, as we regard the clenched fist as the most effective use of the hand as a weapon. However, the open palm is a very dangerous weapon when used by a trained practitioner. It has the advantage too of not being as dangerous to the user. It is much easier to injure the fingers and knuckles when the fist is clenched.

As in Tai Chi Combat the fighting side of Pa-kua makes use of what we can call 'recoil' energy. For instance, if the waist is twisted to the left to send out the right palm, the recoil of the waist – the twist-back of the waist – sends out the left palm with even greater force. This is also true of the Japanese art of Aikido, which we shall come to later. Some students of martial arts believe that the founder of Aikido, Morihei Uyeshiba, found much of his inspiration from the techniques of Pa-kua. Uyeshiba's English language biographer, John Stevens, did not share this view and wrote, 'Since there were no Chinese masters on the same level as Morihei, he likely dismissed, perhaps unjustly, mainland (Chinese) arts as unworthy of serious study.'[10] Such a claim, whilst understandable in a partisan student of Aikido, is not worthy of a second's credence. I do not know of a single empty-handed Japanese martial art which does not owe something to the martial arts of China, and many prestigious martial artists openly express their debt to the Chinese. Even today, Japanese and Okinawan masters visit China, Taiwan and Singapore or Malaysia to learn more.

Pa-kua, Hsing-I and Tai Chi, then, are the Chinese trio of internal arts. They have all been connected with the Eight Trigrams in some way, they all place emphasis on the mind-body relationship, have Taoist connections, rely on Chi power to some extent and continue to attract and delight western students. Of the three, only Tai Chi has become widespread. This is probably due to the long, slow, solo forms of the latter; something which is missing in the other two.

In Chinese language the word 'Chin' means to grab hold of or seize. The word 'Na' means to control or keep hold of. Combined, the two words give us the name of another martial art which is not well known outside the martial arts circles; Chin-na, the art of gripping and holding. Obviously, all martial arts which use only the empty hands have techniques of gripping the body of an opponent, but Chin-na is devoted to the study of such techniques exclusively, and in detail.

In Tai Chi, movements such as Pull, Needle at Sea Bottom and Step Back to Drive Monkey Away can be interpreted as seizing or holding techniques when applied to a partner. Part of a Chin-na student's training is to understand the joints of the body; how they can be twisted and locked. Another part is the study of vital points of the body, and at a deeper level to be aware of the flow by the use of pressure. A third aspect is the study of medicinal herbal remedies so that cures can be brought about for victims of Chin-na attack. When carried to extremes, Chin-na is a gruesome, horror-movie martial art which we do not want to dwell on in a book about Tai Chi!

Some Tai Chi clubs concentrate some of their training time on examining how the body of the partner can be temporarily immobilised or made to 'seize up' for an instant so that an unbalancing push can be given. It also helps solo form training to know something about the joints and the best way of using them. For instance, when the leg is bent in the Bow Stance it is anatomically better for the shin to move down over the foot so that the ankle is not bent to the inside or outside. At one time in his career Cheng Man-ch'ing studied ways of attacking the vital points of the body in anticipation of a challenge that he expected. In the event the challenge never materialised. In common with Tai Chi, Chin-na uses large, medium and small circles for its joint locking techniques. Of great importance also is the development of a powerful grip using variations of finger and thumb; for instance gripping only with the index finger and thumb, index and middle finger and thumb, and so on. In this connection one is reminded of Chen-style master, Chen Fake, who 'practised with a wooden staff about four metres long and fifteen centimetres thick. He shook the heavy thing three hundred times a day as a way to exercise his wrist strength.'[3] Once, when attacked by a man with a spear, Chen gripped the haft of the weapon, gave a slight twist and jabbed the spear back at the man sending him some four metres away. This type of technique is found in the syllabus of Chin-na. If a martial art is to be effective in fighting, it must take into account as many circumstances that might arise as possible. The study of Tai Chi Combat shows that methods akin to those of Chin-na are essential.

Ideally, Tai Chi overcomes an opponent by using his own force, so that any contest is over with the first attack and defensive movement. Though this rarely happens, it is part of the appeal of the art; a superlative and entrancing theory. In the introduction to his translation of Sun Tzu's book, 'The Art of War', Thomas Cleary cites a story about two court physicians. The first one would always notice the faintest symptom of illness and cure his patient without delay, before the symptoms became more dramatic. This physician's reputation never grew. His younger brother dealt with illnesses when there were very noticeable and grave symptoms, and his methods were correspondingly spectacular. His reputation spread far and wide. The ideal of curing an illness almost before it begins was the fundamental idea in Sun Tsu's treatise on warfare, some two thousand years old. It has affinities to the ideal of Tai Chi; of not meeting force with force, of not escalating a conflict, but of curing it at the outset.

Sun Tzu said that the superior general or political leader detects the possibility of conflict before it begins and takes measures to arrest it. If conflict breaks out he finds the best way to end through bargaining. If he cannot end it through bargaining and fighting continues he will find a way to end it with the least possible loss of life, and so on. Always he searches for methods to stop escalation. This is a true Taoist approach to all matters, and it has attracted the attention of politicians, generals and guerrilla fighters for centuries. On a smaller scale it has been studied by martial artists.

One of the passages in 'The Art of War' reads: 'In martial arts, it is important that strategy be unfathomable, that form be concealed, and that movements be unexpected, so that preparedness against them be impossible.' Thus, concealment or secrecy furthers the aim of a rapid conclusion to all conflict. The traditional Chinese practice of concealing methods and theories has been carried to what we in the West would regard as an extreme. It is not unknown for Chinese martial arts teachers to actually show foreigners and outsiders the wrong way to do something so that they will believe they have been taught some sought-after skill when in reality it is worthless. I remember showing a Chinese teacher a movement which I had learned – he nodded, indicating that it was right, but I could tell from his face that he was holding something back.

When a student learns the Tai Chi solo forms it is hard for him to guess how the movements can be applied to combat, at first. This is especially true for those students who have never done a martial art before. Students in this category have no means, except common sense, of verifying whether the applications they have been given will work or not. If everyone in the class has been shown the same thing, they can all go on merrily training at their application techniques, oblivious to the true situation. At the same time it would be a mistake to be overly suspicious of one's teacher's motives and methods. Common sense and a little out-of-class experiment with a willing partner is an acid test.

Although The Art of War goes into detail about fighting terrain, weather conditions for armies and other factors governing the conduct of warfare, the overall intent of the book seems to be to form a new mental attitude in those who read it. Obviously the number of situations which can arise in warfare must be almost infinite, so even if every conceivable instance were listed in such a book a day would dawn in which the inconceivable happens. By having the right attitude of mind a person trained according to the principles of this book would know how to meet even this. The general would understand the principles, the officers the strategy, the non-commissioned officers the tactics, and the men the use of weapons. So, a student of Tai Chi tries to understand the principles of yin and yang in order that his strength and Chi will respond to those principles. He aims to make his whole body follow his Chi so that in every situation the parts of his body will adapt the techniques accordingly. From the large scale to the small the Taoist message of Sun Tzu's book has echoed down the centuries.

Although Aikido is a Japanese martial art it should be dealt with in this book because in the eyes of many martial artists, especially westerners, it has some relationship with Tai Chi, on several levels. The founder of Ai-ki-do (meeting of the Spirit Way) was Morihei Uyeshiba (1883–1969). He was the son of an influential farmer, with samurai ancestors, and the Kumano district where he was born was a traditional centre of Japanese mysticism. In common with other famous martial artists, both before and after him, Uyeshiba was a sickly child. The boy studied the religious texts of Shingon Buddhism, believed fervently in the Shinto gods of the national Japanese faith, and showed an uncommon interest in all religious matters. By subjecting himself to a Spartan way of life which included a daily dousing in ice cold water, Uyeshiba improved his health. He spent some time living in Tokyo but preferred a more rural life and returned to his own village. He had begun to study Jujitsu and found it an absorbing subject. He married, joined the army and studied all manner of martial arts. One practice of his is worth mentioning as it reminds us of training in hard Chi Kung (see Chapter 6).

According to biographer Stevens, Uyeshiba used to pound his skull 'against a stone slab a hundred times a day'. His desire to build up his physical strength and resistance to pain was extraordinary, but in addition to the demands he made on his body, Uyeshiba was equally tormented by spiritual matters. His early life consisted of an endless search for something which he could not define. After some years of this, which took place amidst an eventful outside life, Uyeshiba met the last of the old-time Japanese warriors, Sokaku Takeda. This was a man who feared nothing and no one. With the temperament of a slightly wounded tiger, Takeda was a nineteenth-century Dirty Harry. After Sokaku had given a martial arts demonstration, Uyeshiba met him in a challenge contest. Stevens simply states in sympathetic tones that the future founder of Aikido was 'deftly handled' by Sokaku and thereafter became his pupil.

The martial art Sokaku taught was called Daito Ryu. After a period of close study Uyeshiba once more went his own way. Sokaku, though a fighter without peer, did not have the character to match it, nor the thirst for spiritual fulfilment which spurred his pupil on. Uyeshiba's life story makes enthralling reading and what emerges from it is that he was a man susceptible to visions, capable of very unusual feats, apparently able to read the thoughts of those around him, and possessed of exceptional, irrepressible physical strength and energy. He once had a contest with an accomplished swordsman, an unarmed man against an armed one, and made it impossible for the attacker to strike him. Asked for an explanation of this, he replied that 'Just prior to your attacks, a beam of light flashed before my eyes, revealing the intended direction.' Right after this event, Stevens says that the turning point in Uyeshiba's life occurred. 'Suddenly, Morihei started to tremble and then felt immobilised. The ground beneath his feet began to shake, and he was bathed with rays of pure light streaming down from heaven. A golden mist engulfed his body, causing his petty conceit to vanish . . .'[10]

Although he lived in the twentieth century, the man's life reminds one of the ancient Taoist hermits who pepper the history of Chinese martial arts, performing their seeming miracles, overcoming all attacks and able to move with such speed that they virtually fly. Behind these external accomplishments hovers an invisible wisdom which makes everything possible. In common with Tai Chi masters of the past, Uyeshiba's training was physically severe (again, softness is built on strength). Aikido is an evasive, defensive, soft art compared with Karate or Jujitsu; whether the severe training is essential to such arts or simply commonly found is hard to say. Another interesting point of comparison between Uyeshiba and the Chen family members is that they all came from rural, farming backgrounds. This proximity to nature, in which most Taoist teachings are set, may be important.

What Uyeshiba experienced within himself and expressed in his life itself, his Aikido descendants have expressed in words and diagrams, references to the laws of physics and mechanics, psychology, physiology, mysticism, Hinduism, Buddhism, Shintoism and a veritable shower of ideas connected with such subjects. The techniques of the art themselves are all based on circular, spiral or undulating forms of movement, which in theory at least make yielding in order to counter the order of the day. What some modern exponents have done, and Stevens acknowledges this, is to try to imitate the effortless ease with which the master in later life disposed of his attackers. Often at a demonstration of Aikido, nothing more than a token gesture is made at an attacker and he falls. This, though meant to be a real technique, can produce nothing more than misunderstanding in the minds of the credulous and disbelief in the minds of people with common sense. If a martial art works it must be shown to work, especially in front of the general public; and if it does not work it should not be shown, except as part of a farce, or parody.

More responsible Aikidoka (Aikido students) show their art clearly and point out the necessary reservations which must be made for it as a method of self defence. In my view the two aspects of Aikido which are closest to the art of Tai Chi are the evasive footwork and body shifting, plus the use of the palms for pushing. The arm bending and locking of Aikido as an immediate counter measure I have no time for, because the arms of a fighting man or woman cannot be bent and locked unless he is in such pain or a state of semi-consciousness or drunkenness that he cannot control them; or unless his physical strength is vastly inferior to that of his opponent. Perhaps Uyeshiba could have done these things. In the foot work and body shifting of Aikido through movement after movement there is an echo of the same sweeping and swirling, rising and falling energy which is found in the internal martial arts of China. When moving in this way one experiences a kind of joy and exhilaration of movement which needs no apologia, no analysis and no diagrams.

There are two western systems of postural re-education which should be mentioned in connection with martial art and Tai Chi in particular. This is because they are often spoken of in the same context; that is, ways of moving. They are the Alexander system and the Feldenkrais system. Alexander discovered something akin to the 'letting do' of the Taoists, and Feldenkrais brought together many strands of knowledge concerning posture, joint movement, breathing and psychology.

Alexander was a man who gave dramatic presentations on stage. The condition of his voice was therefore of great importance to him, and when he began to experience difficulty in speaking it was necessary for him to find a remedy for it as soon as possible. He devised many methods, some of them involving the use of mirrors, to find out if, when he was speaking, he did something with his posture which interfered with the production of sound. Each time he thought that he had discovered what he was doing wrong, and corrected it, then some other fault in his posture would appear to replace it. Time passed. He became more engrossed in trying to find out why he could not find the correct posture, particularly the position of his head in relation to his upper spine, than in his career as an elocutionist. After much research on himself he came to the understanding that no matter how much effort he put into correcting his posture using the directions of his mind in guiding his body he could not succeed. If he told himself to move a couple of centimetres this way or that way, or pull back his shoulders or raise his head, it made no difference. Habit, tension, and especially an incorrect picture of his posture, derived from what turned out to be wrongly interpreted sensations of his posture, always overcame his intentions. He realised as the years went by that almost everyone's image of how he or she is standing or moving is in fact wrong.

If you ask an adult to tell you in some detail how he thinks he is standing up, and where his head is in relation to his spine, he will very often get it wrong. He will believe for instance that his shoulders are evenly dropped or level with one another when they are not; that his chin is lowered when it is jutting forward, and so on. Even if you correct this and show him what is wrong in a mirror, within a few seconds he will go back to the old position. Alexander continued his research and used himself mainly as a guinea pig. At last he discovered what he called 'primary control'. This was principally to do with the relationship between the head and the cervical vertebrae, their tension and position, and the finding of a kind of mobile, on-going means of adjusting this relationship in daily life.

To condense his theories: means exist of re-educating some people, but not all, to help themselves to give up old habits of moving and allowing a different part of the nervous system and brain to regulate their movement. For this to be realised, a long period of regular training and dedicated practise is needed, punctuated by refresher visits to a teacher from time to time, to check on progress. Remarkable results have been achieved through the Alexander system. The connection with Tai Chi lies in several areas. One of the sayings of the Tai Chi classics is that the head should be suspended from above, as if held by a hair. For this to happen the neck must be free, not fixed. This freeing of the neck is one of the main focuses of the Alexander system. In Tai Chi the spine should be naturally erect and the centre of gravity lowered. For this to happen the knees have to be slackened from their habitual tension and the sacral and lower lumbar vertebrae must be released from the unnecessary state of backward and upward pressure, caused by wrong muscular tension. This too is one of the results of Alexander training. In many people it results in them becoming a little taller. Today it is not uncommon for Tai Chi and Alexander training to come together from time to time in special seminars.

Feldenkrais was a man of many parts; highly intelligent, sensitive and endlessly interested in the relationship between posture and psychology. One of the subjects which interested him earlier in his career was the role of posture in sexual behaviour; that is, in making love. He found that many people with sexual problems were unable to move the pelvis freely backward and forward. The guilt they felt about sex and the sexual act more or less froze their pelvis on to their upper body. Feldenkrais studied this subject in some detail.

He was also a Judo enthusiast and reached Black Belt standard. When doing Judo, especially in fighting on the floor, the hips, waist and general pelvic area come in for a lot of movement. One can say that in Judo groundwork the lower back must be flexible and free moving for a player to be successful. A Judoka (Judo student) with the same problems as the people with sexual problems would not be able to perform techniques successfully.

Similar things can be said about Tai Chi performance. Waist turning, rippling the waist and pelvis, or making the pelvis undulate when pushing, are all examples of this. Freedom of the scapula or shoulder blade, to which about a dozen muscles are attached, is another example of the crossing of Tai Chi and Feldenkrais paths. Feldenkrais wrote and held seminars about such subjects and gathered a world-wide following. On a Tai Chi and Chi Kung course which I attended some years ago in Boston, a leading Feldenkrais teacher was there helping students with their postural difficulties and giving simple and helpful exercises to correct them.

The subjects broached in this chapter, and many others, are clearly akin to Tai Chi in their several ways. This is because they all contain some kind of fundamental knowledge about the way we work, particularly with regard to how we move. Studying any one of them can throw light on the others and increase our knowledge of ourselves.

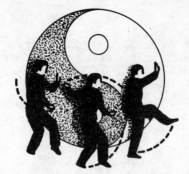

6 · CHI KUNG

In Greek mythology there is a substance called ichor, which flows through the blood vessels of the gods, giving their blood a special quality. The Chinese believe that in addition to the energies in the human body detected by western science there is another energy which they call Chi. It is usually translated as internal energy, and Chi Kung means the cultivation of internal energy.

The study of Chi Kung extends far back in time, beyond the origins of Tai Chi forms. It is carried out by adopting certain postures, regulating the breath and concentrating the mind. Some authorities claim that the practice of Chi Kung can be traced back at least four thousand years to the Yao period. The 'Spring and Autumn Annals' state that people who lived in damp and humid conditions, which led to stagnation of the blood and spirits, were advised to do certain breathing exercises and to perform a kind of dance. During the Warring States period from 770 to 222 BC it was written:

> When you inhale and exhale intentionally, this helps to bring in the fresh air and get rid of the stale air. If you move like a bear and stretch like a bird, this can result in longer life.

These ideas were preserved in the form of carvings on jade and are known as the Chi Kung formula. Further proof of the existence in ancient times of Chi Kung was unearthed in 1979 when a painted relic was found. It showed men and women doing movements in imitation of the movements of animals. It dated from the Western Han dynasty (206 BC–AD 24). In the second century, a famous Chinese doctor, Hua Tuo, wrote that the hinge on a door which is often used will never become covered with insects or infected by them, meaning that exercise and stretching helps to keep the body healthy. He is credited with the invention of a series of movements combined with breathing based on the 'frolics' of the Five Animals: tiger, deer, bear, monkey and bird. The movements are usually known as the Frolics of the Five Animals. Over the next two thousand years references to Chi Kung appear in different surviving writings. It is not surprising therefore that such an ancient, widely accepted and apparently effective system of health cultivation was incorporated into martial arts, including Tai Chi.

If we try to get a little closer to a definition of Chi Kung, or better still of Chi, we come up against a cultural and intellectual gap. In the West we have been subjected to a scientific education and the need for an intellectual proof of the existence of things. We need our famous 'scientific proof' and our 'scientific fact'. If something is described as a scientific fact then in the speaker's mind this is almost the same as saying that God himself gave him the information. Whilst science has its place, scientific fact is not the only criterion; there is such a thing as common sense based on experience.

Recently in a BBC radio food programme a scientist stated that he would get the Nobel Prize for science if he could prove why it is that certain people are sensitive to certain foods – not allergic but sensitive. The fact of the sensitive reaction exists, but the scientific explanation for it does not. Only an idiot would say that the people who experienced this reaction were imagining it. At present we have to take the same attitude towards Chi, its existence and definition. Chi can be thought of as a fine energy which assists and accompanies all the scientifically proven activities of the body and mind: digesting, seeing, homeostasis, thinking, feeling, moving and sensing and so on. Anything which human beings do is assisted at some stage by Chi.

However, there is one misconception which has crept into the thinking of some westerners about Chi, especially in connection with Tai Chi. This is that there is only one type of Chi. This misconception is partly the fault of some teachers, but also the fault of lax research on the part of students, because the information exists in a number of books on traditional Chinese medicine. Every process and every structure and organ in a human being has its own Chi, its own activity-assisting-finer-energy. There are many forms of Chi and the process of cultivating the Chi is not as straightforward as many have assumed. Because the bulk of Tai Chi teachers have concentrated their attention, perhaps mistakenly, on the Chi which is said to accompany the intake, absorption and use of air, the idea has become widespread that this is the only form of Chi. If you are studying a subject and hoping for a quick, easy way through it, it is consoling to simplify what is involved, even if it is a mistake. Chi study is a case in point. If we grant that Chi, vitality, exists, and experience indicates that it does, then we must also grant that it is a subject at least as complex and difficult to understand as the application of western medicine. If books and teachers give a simplified view it is misleading and could even be dangerous.

Everyone now accepts that acupuncture can have beneficial effects. The effects are produced by stimulating or sedating the Chi flow along the invisible channels which run on the surface and interior of the body. In terms of experience we can take this as a sufficient and sound empirical proof of the existence of Chi and leave it at that. Chi exists. At the same time Chi is merely a concept, like Energy. It is only experienced in its variety, not in some pure and pristine state. It is present in many aspects of Chinese culture which can be divided into approximate though overlapping groups.

MEDICINE

The chief medical recognition of Chi lies in the application of fine needles to the acupuncture points, the burning of moxa powder on the same points, the use of massage along the Chi channels, the palpation of the pulses at the wrist to ascertain the quality of Chi in various organs, the relating of foods and herbs to the yin and yang qualities which affect the Chi, the use of medically supervised Chi Kung exercises under controlled conditions for specific ailments and to build up resistance to disease, and the application of needles to produce anaesthesia. As a result of the medical drive to study Chi Kung in China, there are now many colleges, businesses, schools and other organisations where simple Chi Kung exercises are performed in groups. Since 1949 the Chinese medical authorities have carried out extensive and careful tests, accompanied by statistical analysis, in the use of Chi Kung therapy.

Prior to this western-inspired investigation of Chi and the consequent assembling of data, it seems that every specialist in the different disciplines in which it was used would proceed along the lines that he had been taught by his teacher. The need for tables of results was not felt necessary in quite the same way, and proven methods overlapped into folk lore and less easily verifiable beliefs. Nowadays Chinese medicine includes western methods side by side with traditional ones, and presents anyone interested in the history of medical ideas with an enigma. It is as though when we look at the world, the brain does not blend the impressions from our two eyes into one, but presents us with two simultaneous but different pictures of the same subject. What a strange experience that would be. But Chinese physicians seem able to embrace this dual experience comfortably, partly because of the discovery that certain groups of illnesses respond better to western treatment, especially in an emergency, than they do to Chinese; and other groups respond better to Chinese traditional treatment, with Chi as a background. As the Chinese turn their attention and aspirations more towards the West, it has become more common for martial-arts teachers to cite the accumulated western-style proof of the usefulness of Chi Kung as a recommendation for the Chi Kung found in their training.

MARTIAL ARTS

If we take styles of fighting which we are familiar with in the West, such as boxing, wrestling and even the Sumo tournaments which have become popular in recent years, we recognise the obvious fact that certain contestants have a clear superiority over the rest. Mike Tyson as heavyweight boxing champion and the really amazing skill of Mohammed Ali in his early years are good examples. Chinese martial artists would say that the Chi of these two men was high, in the particular skill they had chosen. Even without hearing about Chi, Tyson and Ali have cultivated it. Theirs is hard Chi, and the Chi Kung they have, so to speak, unwittingly followed is Hard Chi Kung. The training method followed by Morihei Uyeshiba of banging his head against a stone slab falls within this definition too, as is the regular running of Sun Lu-t'ang holding on to the tail of a horse. Hard Chi is Chi which has been concentrated in the muscles and given them extra toughness and power. Soft Chi is the Chi used in Tai Chi, Pa-kua and their offshoots, to increase sensitivity, lightness, agility and also power, but a form different to the power of Hard Chi.

CIRCUS ACTS

Under this heading we can put the cultivation of Chi for no other reason than display purposes which have no practical use. For instance, some men have shown feats such as lying down on a bed or on broken glass and having a slab of stone placed on their abdomen which is then smashed by a sledge hammer. Such spectacles have been seen all over the world and have drawn many 'oohs' and 'aahs' from audiences, but little else.

ARTS WORLD

By cultivating the Chi, mainly through the use of breath, painters, musicians, actors and calligraphers have been able to produce works and skills which are said not to be possible without the Chi.

OCCULT ARTS AND SECRET SOCIETIES

A large body of literature exists on the use of Chi cultivation to obtain supernormal experiences, flashes of insight, psychic powers, healing at a distance, injuring one's foes at a distance, attaining immortality, being impervious to poisons, and so on. To such areas belong people who advocate the use of Chi Kung to acquire strange sexual powers. This is a very misty world of Chi Kung and, where it has touched Tai Chi theory, it has done more harm than good.

RELIGIOUS WAYS

The use of Chi Kung appears in Taoist religion, Ch'an Buddhism and in some minor Chinese sects which have appeared from time to time. This is again a misty area of the subject. In the case of Taoism a distinction should be made and remembered between the religion and the philosophical way. The religion had its priests, its hierarchy, its tenets of faith and rituals, combined with instructions on the use of Chi to obtain religious experience. The philosophy pointed towards a way of being in accord with Nature, of letting the Chi flow and be as it was meant to be. Ch'an Buddhism, Zen, has something in common with this approach.

These several worlds in which Chi Kung is found all influenced thinking about Tai Chi, its teaching and development. Students who study Tai Chi may find that it is useful to know something about these other influences so that when they meet them they will be able to identify their origin and assess how seriously or otherwise they want to take them. Let us look at them in more detail.

MEDICINE

One of the chief causes of illness, according to traditional Chinese medicine, is stagnant Chi or stasis. For instance, a case of poor blood circulation might be diagnosed as connected with weak Chi of the blood, causing a slowing down of its movement and failure to penetrate fully into all the tiny blood vessels. On a mental level one could say that stagnant Chi contributes to the syndrome of worrying continually about the same problem; mental stasis.

Chi Kung therapy has cured many complaints. Among them are gastric and duodenal ulcers, headaches, poor eye sight, stomach ache, neurasthenia and spastic colon. The therapy stimulated or evened out the flow of Chi and the body was able to return to normal. Cases also exist in which the diagnosis by a western physician differed from that of a Chinese one; duodenal ulcer was the western choice and dysfunction of the stomach and spleen the Chinese. Other cases have been cited in which neither western nor other traditional Chinese treatments were effective but Chi Kung therapy was. The key to such cures is very often simply a matter of doing the exercises prescribed! They are not difficult to learn but some patients do not have the tenacity to keep at them on a regular basis.

The therapy is divided into two parts: static and dynamic. In static Chi Kung a number of different postures are adopted; standing still, leaning, sitting, squatting, lying back and lying down. In the dynamic therapy different postures, one after the other, are carried out, some of them designed to improve the general health and others aimed at specific ailments. An ancillary therapy is Chi Kung self massage or using the hands to direct the Chi. An example of the latter is to place the hands on the abdomen near the navel and make circles around a particular point. In certain Tai Chi teachings the navel or a place just below it, the Tan T'ien, is described as a focal point for the Chi; a point at which the centre of gravity can be established so that one's balance is not easily disturbed.

We find here an obvious relationship between the two subjects and can surmise that on the basis of the respective ages of the two that Tai Chi took its ideas from Chi Kung, and not the other way round. Those who promote Chi Kung in China today seem to regard Tai Chi as nothing more than one of the many forms of Chi Kung. Though this may be true in a certain sense, Tai Chi has developed so much into an independent subject that a clear distinction has to be made. An analogy for us could be European dancing. Dancing may at one time have been mainly folk dancing, but over the centuries it has diversified so much that for example we would not call classical ballet by that name.

The Frolics of the Five Animals mentioned earlier are today classified as part of Chi Kung therapy. A saying associated with these movements is that one should move as if playing with waves and currents while the mind soars over the sea. The Chinese physician, Hua Tuo, who is credited with inventing the Five Animals Frolics, was possibly laying future foundations of Hsing-I in which twelve animal forms are taught. In the names of Tai Chi postures, as we have seen, the presence of animals is not uncommon: White Crane, Snake Creeps Down and Tame Tiger. The Frolics are movements based on those of the Bear, Crane, Deer, Tiger and Monkey. When they are performed, not only has the Chi to flow in the prescribed manner and the body replicate the movements, but the bearing and general demeanour of the student should convey the spirit and feeling of the animal concerned. The characteristics of the Frolics are:

Mind and body working together
Flexible, spiralling and circular movements
Slow movements and fast movements. Slow 'like spinning silk' and fast 'like a frightened snake'
Appreciation of weight, stability and subtlety
Softness and hardness to appear according to the type of movement
Breathing to be in harmony with movement
Persevering and conscientious practice

We can say that if we take the whole spectrum of Tai Chi then these same characteristics can be applied to it also. When the Frolics are performed the student tries to see inside the animal and catch its spirit. For instance, although the bear is heavy and lumbering and in some senses awkward, it is nevertheless quick and agile when it has to be. These qualities must be 'carried' in the student as he trains and he must repeatedly bring them into his movements. The crane flies as if it were 'playing with clouds and the moon' yet it also stands 'as tranquil as a pine tree'. The deer leaps and darts but is also very relaxed. The tiger has powerful claws (tense the fingers) and its eyes are filled with power; its movements should 'suggest as hurricane' but also 'contain the quietude of the moon'. The monkey, though playful and constantly busy, nevertheless has its own kind of stillness and in the legend of Monkey has tremendous power when it uses its magical staff for fighting. So the Five Frolics are much more varied and versatile than the type of Tai Chi we generally see in the West. Their moods change markedly compared with the mood of Tai Chi which emphasises stillness and a kind of quiet dignity; slow and measured. It is only when we come to some of the older forms of Tai Chi, as we have noted, and their application to combat, that we find closer links with the Five Frolics.

The other aspect of Chi Kung therapy which is sometimes taught in

Tai Chi classes or introduced as part of the warming up or warming down exercises is self massage. We have all experienced banging an elbow or knee and instinctively placing a hand on it. This is partly to touch the spot and find out what has happened but also we 'believe', without putting it into words, that we will 'make it better'. Mothers comfort fallen children with their hands. Western spiritual healers make passes with their hands over the sick bodies of their patients. This widespread belief in the healing power of the hands has been extended in some detail in Chi Kung therapy. Some therapists claim that it has become a science. The techniques of the hands which are used are similar to those of western medical massage and are:

> Patting with the palm, tapping with the tips of the fingers, stroking with the palm, twisting, poking, pressing, kneading, pinching, rubbing, chopping, seizing and pounding.

In fact the actions are very similar to the hitting methods of martial arts; just the manner of using the hand and the intention are different. In short, any way in which the human hand can be used has been adopted. In some cases, chop sticks, bamboo and padded sticks are applied instead of the hands. The chief difference between western massage and Chi Kung massage, whether administered by oneself or by another person, is in the detailed focus of the hand and the theory behind it; the following is an example of this. Sometimes the orbit of the eyeball is massaged. The orbit itself is divided up into areas which are supposed to be related to the organs of the body. This therapy is sometimes called Acupressure, and indeed follows similar but coarser lines to Acupuncture. Additionally, acupressure has stroking and tapping movements along the Chi channels of the body. In some Tai Chi classes these types of movement are taught for self administration, to loosen up the body, dispel tension and try to bring the centre of gravity down, clearing the thoughts.

One of the important aspects of Chi Kung therapy, according to my information, is the amount of time which has to be devoted to it, and the large number of repetitions needed to produce lasting results. The 'Five Minutes A Day' formula to bring you beauty, health and strength, so beloved of western book publishers and holders of seminars on such subjects, does not apply to Chi Kung therapy. Reports from China indicate that periods of practice begin with whatever the patient can sustain without exhausting him or her, and can then extend up to eight hours where serious diseases are involved. One should also bear in mind that this is supervised therapy with medical instruments at hand to monitor irregularities in heart, lung and blood pressure and so on. This is no 'trip' in the amphetamine sense but a whole-hearted attempt to become physically sound and strong. It reminds us of the hard training undergone by some Tai Chi students.

The 'circus' acts of Chi Kung in the West date, in any appreciable sense, from the early 1970s when a Chinese martial arts troupe visited the United States for the first time since the Second World War. In addition to the beautiful and dramatic displays of martial skills that they gave, one man, Hou Shuying, broke a granite slab with his head. He apparently suffered no ill effects! The feat set the martial arts world talking. They had seen karate men break wood and tiles but this was something else. Any strong or courageous person can punch and break a suitable piece of wood but it needs something special to break granite with your head. Another troupe visited London and gave a display at the Albert Hall. Their feats included lying on broken glass, the head covered with a concrete slab which was then broken with a sledge hammer. The man with the concrete-proof head got up and seemed none the worse for wear. Some time later at the Great Wall restaurant in Chinatown, London, two more martial artists from China demonstrated unusual power in the neck. They each took a strong spear which was tested by the ever-cynical members of the Press who were there in large numbers and placed the point against their necks. By resting the blunt end of the spear on the floor they bent the haft of each spear to breaking point, without any sign of injury. These amazing activities are carried out not only by fully grown men but also by little children, which means that they do not depend solely on strength or hardness of the bone. Although children's bones do contain more soft tissue than an adult's bones, one cannot put the feats down to mere pliability of the bones in these cases. It has been suggested that they are tricks, that they are merely the clever use of mechanics, that the body has been specially hardened by medicines and so forth. The performers themselves say it is the result of Chi Kung training.

In Tai Chi circles attitudes to these acts varies. Some instructors have personal 'turns' which they pull out of the hat on special occasions; others do not concern themselves with such things. The chief characteristic of these 'mysteries' of the East is that they are of no practical value at all. They are not even useful for fighting, because a demonstration is set up and a real fight is not. The person suffering the blow has had time to prepare himself, set his body and focus his Chi. The man with the sledge hammer uses it in a particular way, at the correct angle and so on. In a fast moving fight, if the man with the sledge hammer had hit the performer on the head with it then the story might have ended up in quite a different way. A favourite feat of Tai Chi teachers who give demonstrations of special skills is to ask several members of the audience to stand behind one another and try to push him over. They almost never succeed. But the position is a static one and it can be seen that the mechanics of the forces at play make it hard for the audience members to succeed. In Push Hands of course, if the fur was flying, this static skill would be of no use.

ARTS WORLD

In the world of art forms the beauty of Chinese dancing is due in part to the use of Chi Kung. In the *Spring and Autumn Annals* there is a chapter devoted to ancient music. This work, which is about 2,300 years old, relates how dances were devised to increase the fitness of the people. During the same period, dances were produced using the then current weapons of war. Other dances based on animal movements, dances performed in honour of the gods, dances of exorcism and shaman dances all have this awareness of the existence of Chi power running through them.

Chang Chung-yan, in his book *Creativity and Taoism*, wrote: 'We find that the great masters of painting make their contributions only when they . . . dwell in a state of inner serenity.' Later in the same book he says that 'When Su Tung-p'o holds the brush he feels that potentialities issue forth like spring water from the ground. . . .' In Chang Huai's 'Treatise on Painting', quoted by Chang Chung-yuan, we find that 'His brush will secretly be in harmony with movement and quiescence and all forms will issue forth.' This idea of inner serenity and the release of potentialities through the brush, of being in harmony with movement, yang, and quiescence, yin, are part and parcel of the gentle use of Chi, harmonising with Chi. They are also to be found in Tai Chi forms.

Tai Chi is sometimes called meditation in movement but it could equally be called painting in movement, since both the painter and student of the form rely on similar factors. The movement of Tai Chi is carried out against a background of inner stillness, and the movement and life of a Chinese painting owes much to the presence of a stillness in the open spaces of the picture contrasting with the action of a figure or wind-swept tree, or the stillness of a 'rooted' mountain contrasting with the motion of a bird in flight. These forms of Chi Kung are a far cry from breaking granite with one's head.

OCCULT ARTS AND SECRET SOCIETIES

China has always been a country of secret societies, and many of them had practices which can be called occult in a very general sense. The variety of these practices cannot be covered in a book which is mainly about Tai Chi but there is one idea found in many of them which can be an axis for all. This is the idea that matter and energy can be transformed, not only in the ways which we can observe and which western science has discovered: the seasons, the digestion of food, the activity of the sun itself, and so on. This central idea maintains that matter and energy can be transformed by magical rites, by chanting, by meditation and other methods. The transformation takes place both in the physical and 'psychic' worlds.

From the point of view of Chinese thought, the internal energies and substances of man, of which Chi is one example, are undergoing immense changes in ordinary life. Certain of the practices I have mentioned aim to bring about different transformations from those of ordinary life, by manipulating internal energy. Broadly speaking, Chinese thought sees human beings containing the following substances and energies:

CHI:

Normal forms of Chi come from the parents at the moment of conception (yuan chi), sometimes called Pre-birth or Pre-natal Chi; from food, the digestion of which produces Grain Chi (ku-chi); from the air which we breathe into the lungs which produces Natural Air Chi (kung-chi). The latter gives us the expression Chi Kung. Pre-natal Chi is what is said to give a human being his or her constitution. It is stored in the kidneys, which also in Chinese thought are closely connected with sexual energy. When these three forms of Chi begin to circulate throughout the body they produce what is called Normal Chi. Normal Chi keeps us warm, deals with the Fluids and Blood described below, protects us from pernicious external influences, helps us to move, think, have emotions and feelings. For all these purposes and functions it is differentiated in the body. Chi is said to have four movements: it descends, it rises, it enters and it leaves. When the Chi fails to function correctly, disharmony occurs. It is the purpose of Chi Kung to help this function to be restored.

BLOOD:

When food begins to digest in the body the spleen is said to produce a fine energetic essence which ascends and circulates to the lungs. As it ascends it meets the nourishing or nutritive type of Chi – the two energies interact – and from this meeting the Blood is produced. This is not just the red blood which we in the West think of as blood, but all the qualities of blood as well. The Chi of the heart and lungs then send the Blood around the body. This interdependence of the Chi and Blood is underlined by the fact that the Blood nourishes the organs from which the Chi is produced.

CHING:

Ching is also present at birth along with Chi. Ching is concerned with the way in which a person grows up and develops. This type of Ching is called Pre-natal Ching. Post-natal Ching comes from pure food, that is, food which has been purified by the digestive process. Together with Chi, Ching watches over the rise and fall of one's vitality from cradle to grave; Shakespeare's Seven Ages of Man might have been a description of the operation of Ching. When Ching is defective one can see such things as the failure to mature physically, mentally or emotionally, growing old before one's time and problems with normal sexual functioning.

SHEN:

This is the most difficult of energies to define. The word 'spirit' has often been used to translate Shen. Absence of sound Shen results in insanity, extremes of violence and depression, inner confusion, lack-lustre appearance. The presence of sound Shen brings clarity, a feeling of being in tune with life, a sense of harmony with other people.

FLUIDS:

These are substances such as urine, sweat and saliva. They lubricate the body and come from the digestion of food. They help the work of the Chi and are helped by it.

In order of descent from yang to yin qualities we have Shen, Ching, Chi, Blood and Fluids. It is these substances and energies which the different occult streams of Chinese life have sought to engage and manipulate for a host of different purposes.

RELIGIOUS WAYS

From the point of view of Taoist philosophy, a man of Tao who tries to follow the Taoist Way is one who tries to understand and harmonise with natural energies through movement and stillness. But the Taoist religion is more akin to the occult stream just discussed. Whatever form the religion took in the past, today there are many claiming to teach the Taoist religion employing methods which involve breaking into the natural order and hierarchy of energy transformation for a number of reasons, some of them purely commercial.

One of the energies which is focused on is sexual energy and the Ching and Chi associated with it. Methods exist of stimulating sexual energy and desire in obvious ways such as touching the sexual organs, imagining sexual activities and in less obvious ways connected with posture, breathing and concentration. The idea is that sexual essence can be transformed and used to bring spiritual enlightenment, longevity or even immortality, levitation, the ability to fly, the acquisition of such weight that no one can budge you, and other powers. There is a whole corpus of Chinese literature, most of it couched in symbolic language (Jade Stem equals penis), dealing with such things.

Any student of Tai Chi may come across references to these things which to me means that at some time or other Tai Chi was, so to speak, put in a big sack along with them and given a good shake. When everything was emptied out again a number of fragments of these ideas still stuck to it. In my view, the point is that it is better to leave these matters alone and focus on movement, relaxation and correct form and bear in mind the type of Chi Kung which we will now come back to.

Harking back to the Zen abbot Takuan, and the letter he wrote to Yagyu about swordsmanship, we find a kind of Chi Kung which is more akin to that of the Chinese painters. He was speaking about the mind's tendency to 'stop' or stick to what it perceived. Later he enlarges his theme and says,

When I look at a tree, I perceive one of its leaves is red, and my mind 'stops' with this leaf. When this happens, I see just one leaf and fail to take cognisance of the innumerable other leaves of the tree . . . But when the mind moves on without 'stopping', it takes up hundreds of thousands of leaves without fail. When this is understood we are Kwannons (enlightened beings).[6]

The Chi Kung at work here is subtle, requiring hard work, preparation and long study of oneself, with a teacher. For Tai Chi students it gives a picture of the uninterrupted doing of the forms or Push Hands with a perfect balance between movement and stillness. Takuan goes on to say that once the swordsman has become fully matured in the doctrine of no-mindedness (no-mind-stopping-ness) he is in a sense just as innocent of sword technique as he was before he ever saw or heard of a sword. Yet now of course he has changed.

> Though not consciously trying to
> guard the rice fields from intruders,
> the scarecrow is not after all standing
> to no purpose.[6]

(Bukkoku Kokushi, 1241–1316)

Takuan cites the above poem to illustrate a point. Later he makes another important statement: 'The understanding of principle alone cannot lead one to the mastery of movements of the body and its ways . . . training in detailed technique is not to be neglected.' But the principle of no stopping of the mind should lead. The three stages of beginner in innocence and ignorance, student full of knowledge and effort, swordsmaster in a state of no-mind, show what I would call the sane approach to Chi Kung, the one followed by Taoist philosophers, and by the purest Tai Chi teachers. Even though the student is full of knowledge and technical tricks, he has his teacher with him to keep reminding him of the aim of no-mind; that his swordplay should not ultimately depend on technique alone. This state of affairs guards him from being side-tracked into the type of avenues promulgated by what is left of the Taoist religion and its associated methods.

The Tai Chi counterparts of sword use are the movements of the forms and the training in Push Hands and Tai Chi Combat. By pursuing the aim of no-mind under the guidance of a teacher, a student *is* refining his Chi, *is* doing Chi Kung. It is enough to search repeatedly for relaxation and inner centring, which will lead to no-mind. It is not necessary to clutter up the mind with literally hundreds of theories and practices connected with the Taoist religion, especially when they are learned from books; this leads to everything-in-the-mind, not no-mind.

Fung Yu-lan writes of a tradition which is not widely known but which is relevant to what we are looking at here. It seems that in addition to all the recorded teachings of the Buddha, and the mountain of texts and doctrines which have accumulated in his name, there was a secret teaching which was separate from all the rest. The Buddha passed this teaching to one disciple. It was transmitted orally from one man to another until it reached Bodhidharma, the twenty-eighth Patriarch. Between 520 and 526 AD Bodhidharma travelled to China and founded the Ch'an Buddhist school, in conditions which had already been prepared by Chinese Buddhists. Since that time to the present day a current of teaching whose original source was the secret doctrine of the Buddha has invigorated the cultural life of China, Japan and to some extent the rest of the world. This invigorating stream found some expression in the letter written by Takuan, and, if it were needed, gives added weight to the no-mind approach to Chi Kung.

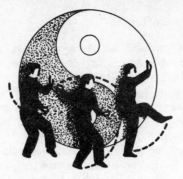

7 · TAI CHI AND I-CHING, YIN-YANG THEORY, FIVE ELEMENTS

The first part of this chapter will attempt to make clear a number of important points about the history of the I-Ching, the Five Element theory and the idea of Yin and Yang. Their relationship with Tai Chi will come in the second part. Dividing the chapter in this way has been necessary because there are a number of misconceptions in the minds of many Tai Chi students about these relationships; misconceptions which at one time I shared. So in order to clarify these it was thought better to give readers a picture based on the writings of scholars and medical writers, rather than repeat the unclear information which is found in many books on Tai Chi. In this way, readers will go into the second half of the chapter better informed, with a better view of the Five Element theory for instance, which will enable them to appraise once again much that they may have read about it already. In writing this chapter I have had to put on one side any feelings of respect I may have for different writers and teachers of Tai Chi, and examine what they wrote and said quite separately from their ability in the art itself.

According to Chinese tradition, the basis for the book which we know as the I-Ching or Book of Changes was laid down by Fu Hsi. Fu Hsi is referred to as the first legendary ruler of China, and his dates are usually given as 2852–2738 BC. He is also given the title of 'subduer of animals, inventor of nets and snares for fishing'. Whether Fu Hsi actually existed and did the things spoken about is irrelevant to Chinese thought. What is important is that such a great and wise ancestor is there in Chinese culture, even today, because it gives us a clue to everything that followed. What followed is that Chinese thought continued to look back, to revere the past and time and again try to ally itself with the past, whatever intellectual contortions were necessary to do so.

After Fu Hsi laid the basis of the I-Ching there was silence for the space of about one thousand years. Tradition does not say anything about this period of the I-Ching's history. During the Shang dynasty (1766–1123 BC) scholars give two different versions of what happened to it. Some maintained that the I-Ching was invented by King Wen (1184–1135 BC) and the more modern scholars adhere to the theory that neither Fu Hsi nor King Wen had anything to do with it. This latter theory points out that during the Shang dynasty there was a method of divination which 'consisted of applying heat to a shell or bone, and then, according to the cracks that resulted, determining the answer to the subject of divination'.[1] It is not a facetious comparison to liken this method of reading the future to that of examining tea leaves left in a cup. Both processes have their random aspect and both depend on the arrangement of visible material. Of course the difference is that divination in China at that period was a much more serious affair than tea leaf reading is today. It would be a mistake to think that because people placed importance on the cracks appearing in shell or bones that they were 'primitive' or 'superstitious' or 'backward' in some way, and not as capable as we are. One can bear in mind that during this dynasty works of art and craft associated with religion were made, and the 'art of this period ... found its highest and most perfect expression in the famous ceremonial bronzes'. The people of the Shang dynasty 'came at the end of a complex artistic evolution and demonstrate a completely mature and developed culture'. There appears on these bronzes the image of a dragon, which gives one some idea of the antiquity of the mythical beast which was used to name some of the Chen style postures of Tai Chi.

During this period, tribes of Tibetan and Turkish immigrants moved into the present Shensi province and founded the Chou state. The worship of the heavens, stars and sun was prominent in their religion and may have contributed to the hierachical view of the universe which is found in the I-Ching. In 1122 BC the Chou dynasty replaced the Shang and lasted until 249 BC. It is said that during the Chou steps were taken to make the traditional divination process clearer. Fung Yu-lan writes that 'such cracks, however, might assume an indefinite number of varying configurations, and so it was difficult to interpret them according to any fixed formula'. It is believed that during the early Chou the oracle bones were set aside in favour of a method using stalks of a plant called milfoil, referred to in later times as yarrow stalks. A fixed number of stalks were used in a certain order and yielded various combinations so that a codified series of interpretations could be drawn up.

Scholars believe that the stalks of the milfoil were the basis for the lines of the I-Ching. At its outset the book was a collection of linear signs. There were only two types of line. One was an unbroken straight line, and the other a line of equal length, divided into two equal parts. At first the lines were arranged in groups of three, one line on top of the other, in different series, to give the Eight Trigrams. Depending on which series emerged during the process of divination the I-Ching could be consulted and the verdict given. Once again there is no information about the earliest development of this method. We can only assume that from the early interpretations some of them became the accepted and traditional ones and the rest were discarded.

Gradually, a picture emerges of a book which grew and spread both in content and influence until it is said that Confucius (551–479 BC) expressed the wish that if he could live for another hundred years he would like to spend fifty of them studying the I-Ching. During the later part of the Chou dynasty but before the time of Confucius the official Eight Trigrams were combined into groups of six lines, to give sixty-four hexagrams and interpretations. A leading Russian researcher into the I-Ching, Iulian K. Shchutskii, gives weight to the idea that the I-Ching had more than one author by pointing out that the book is heterogeneous in content.[12]

Later, another large contribution was made to the book and took the form of appendices called the Ten Wings. This is an important point because it is only in the Ten Wings that we find references to Yin and Yang. It seems that the introduction of Yin-Yang theory as such into I-Ching interpretation was a later event. Prior to it, the Yin-Yang school of thought apparently existed separately; we shall come back to this point, in connection with Tai Chi.

During the Han dynasty (202 BC–AD 220) 'the Yin-Yang concept was also developed by Han scholars in their interpretations of the I-Ching'.[13] During this period 'the first two of the I-Ching's eight basic trigrams (which are) the trigrams of Heaven (ch'ien) and earth (k'un) were equated with Yang and Yin respectively, so that these two metaphysical forces, Heaven and earth, male and female, became the father and mother of all the other trigrams, and in turn, of all creation. Themselves springing from the Great Ultimate (T'ai Chi), they produce by their interaction all the phenomena of the world'. Believers in this thesis saw the trigrams and hexagrams as representations in symbolic form of everything in creation. One should bear in mind that this thesis comes over two thousand five hundred years after the supposed creation of the I-Ching by Fu Hsi and about one thousand five hundred years after the supposed appearance of the I-Ching during the Shang dynasty. The introduction of the Yin-Yang concept into I-Ching interpretation showed those who consulted it that there was danger in going to extremes. This is said to have guided their thinking and action towards the ideal of a golden mean; nothing too much of anything.

From the early centuries of the Christian period up to the present time a multitude of interpretations and uses of the I-Ching have been made. The power and vagueness of the book attracts, confuses, enlightens and delights its devotees. Because the Yin-Yang concept is shared also by the Taoist religion and philosophy, all three streams, originally quite separate, of I-Ching, Yin-Yang and Taoism, have appeared in Tai Chi theory. Before leaving the I-Ching for a moment we should see some of the trigrams and hexagrams, together with examples of their interpretation.

stand for Heaven, father – described in later times as three Yang, masculine lines

stand for earth, mother – described in later times as three Yin, feminine lines

when brought together into one hexagram the two trigrams mean Standstill or Stagnation

A hexagram can be seen from one point of view as consisting of two trigrams, one on top of the other. Shchutskii writes: 'In the theory of the Book of Changes the lower trigram is customarily regarded as referring to the internal life, to what is coming, to what is being created, and the upper trigram to the external world, to what is receding, to what is dissolving'. In the hexagram for Standstill shown above, the yang is diminishing and the yin is increasing. Leaving aside the traditional interpretations of the I-Ching we could see this hexagram of two trigrams as a picture of the increasing role of women in our society and the diminishing role of men!

Finally, the lines were each given a number, starting from the bottom line, from one to six. For divinatory purposes, different attributes were allocated to each line. One such, quoted by Shchutskii, is as follows:

Line 6 represents the Head
Line 5 the Shoulders
Line 4 the Torso
Line 3 the Thighs
Line 2 the Shins
Line 1 the Feet

If taken in a completely literal sense, such an equation of parts of the body with the lines of the hexagrams could be the basis of a relationship between the I-Ching and a complete system of martial arts; a kind of open season on the I-Ching. Let's leave the last word in this section to Joseph Needham, the world famous authority on Chinese history and culture:

'The key word in Chinese thought is *Order* and above all *Pattern* ... Things behave in particular ways not necessarily because of prior action or impulsions of other things, but because their positions in the ever-moving cyclical universe was such that they were endowed with intrinsic natures which made that behaviour inevitable for them ...[14]

The changing picture presented by the sixty-four hexagrams is an ideal expression of the above. The position of a line in the hexagram determines its pathway or direction; its intrinsic nature, broken or unbroken, makes its behaviour inevitable and its relationship with the other lines modifies both its direction and the expression of its nature.

The Yin-Yang concept was developed by early Chinese cosmologists. Their thinking gave rise to the Yin-Yang Chia or Yin-Yang school. The word Yin originally referred to the dark side of a hill or mountain where the sun did not reach, and the word Yang to the light side illuminated by the sun. It is not known when these terms were first used in connection with Chinese explanations of the origin and growth of the universe. According to the classification of Chinese schools made by Ssu-ma T'an in the second century BC, the Yin-Yang Chia was separate from the Tao-Te Chia or School of the Way and its Power, which was the early school of Taoist philosophy. During the

Han dynasty, before the Christian era, the Yin-Yang concept attracted a great deal of attention. People using the I-Ching for divination found in the two words some new inspiration. Richard Wilhelm wrote:

> 'By transference the two concepts were applied to the light and dark sides of a mountain or river . . . Thence the two expressions were carried over into the Book of Changes and applied to the two alternating primal states of being . . . the terms Yin and Yang do not occur in the derived sense either in the actual text of the book or in the oldest commentaries'.[15]

The meaning of the two words gradually widened from that of two primal creative forces to mean such things as: (Yin) 'cold, rest, responsiveness, passivity, darkness, interiority, downwardness, inwardness and decrease', and (Yang) 'heat, stimulation, movement, activity, excitement, vigour, light, exteriority, upwardness, outwardness and increase'. (See *Chinese Medicine – the Web that has no Weaver*, Ted Kaptchuk.[16]) The Yin-Yang concept and the I-Ching exerted a reciprocal action on one another's interpretation.

Since, to state the obvious, we distinguish between things by observing their distinctions and assemble things by observing their similarities, the concept of Yin and Yang can be an amazingly useful tool for analysing many types of activity. As Ted Kaptchuk points out, though, the two words can be misleading unless it is borne in mind that they do not describe fixed states. Both are continually changing because of the action of the one upon the other or rather because the activity of the one evokes the activity of the other. The appeal of such a concept to the Taoists was strengthened by the fact that Taoism has no explicit idea of a Creator. Their interest lies, as Joseph Needham pointed out, in order and patterns of events. In the title of Kaptchuk's book we have a graphic illustration of this; there is a web but no weaver. The universe can be seen as a gigantic interplay of Yin and Yang. Within each Yin there is some Yang to be found and within each Yang some Yin. This division proceeds to infinity.

The concept does have an empirical basis in Chinese traditional medicine, where it has been tested for centuries. A high fever represents a Yang condition, and a state of cold shock a Yin condition. When a patient is in a state of high fever 'he may be in danger of suddenly going into a state of shock'.[16] This piece of medical knowledge echoes the ancient statement of philosophy that when Yang reaches a certain stage of expansion it can go no further and the process begins to return to Yin. The organs of the body are classified into the two divisions and treated accordingly.

Yin	Yang
Heart	Small intestine
Lungs	Large intestine
Pericardium	Stomach
Spleen	Gall Bladder
Liver	Bladder
Kidneys	Triple Burner (not an organ in itself but a relationship between organs)

The most famous Chinese medical treatise is the Nei Ching Su Wen which is known in English as The Yellow Emperor's Book of Internal Medicine. The date of its composition is unknown, and the very existence of the Yellow Emperor, Huang Ti, is in doubt. It is first mentioned in the Annals of the Former Han Dynasty, (206 BC–AD 25). An excellent reference in English is *The Yellow Emperor's Book of Internal Medicine*.[17] Within this book the Yin-Yang concept, the Five Element theory, and the concept of Chi all appear. To my knowledge there is no mention of the I-Ching. Readers are advised to go through this book if they wish to gain an impression of the way these ideas are threaded into the diagnosis, treatment and prevention of disease, and at the same time appreciate the harmonious way in which this is done.

The diagram used by the Chinese to express the Yin-Yang concept at the place of the Supreme Ultimate is shown below. It is the diagram of the 'two fishes', one white and one black with 'eyes' of the opposite colour. Black stands for Yin and white for Yang. The eyes indicate that in the phenomenal world neither aspect exists in its pure form but always contains something of its opposite. Wilhelm wrote that the diagram of the Supreme Ultimate presented speculations of a 'gnostic-dualistic character (which) is foreign to the I-Ching; what it

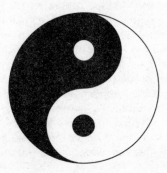

posits is simply the ridge-pole, the line'.[15] It was the brush of Chou Tun-yi, the first 'cosmological philosopher' (1017–1073) which first gave the diagram the name T'ai-chi T'u or Diagram of the Supreme Ultimate: 'The Supreme Ultimate through movement produces Yang. This Movement, having reached its limit, is followed by Quiescence, and by this Quiescence it produces the Yin.'

Fung Yu-lan records that

> Long before this time, some of the religious Taoists (not philosophers) had prepared a number of mystic diagrams as graphic portrayals by which they believed a properly initiated individual could gain immortality. Chou Tun-yi is said to have come into possession of one of these diagrams, which he thereupon reinterpreted and modified into a diagram of his own, designed to illustrate the process of cosmic evolution.'[1]

What many modern western students of Tai Chi believe they have inherited as a composite system, whose most memorable and salient symbols and ideas apparently complement and explain one another, was originally derived from several sources, at different times and places. Personally, I find this an important and memorable point. This is because when one hears of and accepts an idea, symbol or concept, the importance and wisdom of it is difficult to judge, unless one knows something of its history, or has the insight to do so. This is particularly true of us westerners who are not experts in Chinese thought, when we find ourselves confronted with the so-called philosophy of Tai Chi. We are apt to give equal importance to every idea we hear about, not being in a position to evaluate it correctly. This particularly applies to our third subject, the Five Element Theory.

The Chinese word Hsing means to act or to do. Wu is the word for five, and so Wu Hsing means the Five Activities, the Five Things Which Are Being Done. The expression is found in the Book of History, Shou Ching, compiled by Confucius. Though traditionally given a date or origin some two thousand years BC by men who wished to confer the respectability of great age upon it, modern scholarship places the Wu Hsing theory some time in the third or fourth centuries BC The crucial point about this theory is the number Five. In the earliest writings we find references to Five Functions, for instance, and Five Indications, further divided into Five Favourable Indications and Five Unfavourable. Why the number Five was deemed so important I have been unable to find out; why not three or seven?

Fung Yu-lan says that, in the early stages, the Wu Hsing theory was still 'crude'. When the author wrote about them, he was 'still thinking in terms of the actual substances, water, fire, etc., instead of the abstract forces bearing these names, as the Wu Hsing came to be regarded later on.'[1] The Wu Hsing was developed by the Yin-Yang Chia in the thinking about 'the mutual influence between nature and man' and represents a simple scientific attempt to explain the universe's activity. It was a later phase of the Yin-Yang Chia which stated that the interaction of Yin and Yang produces the Five Activities.

In most English translations of the expression Wu Hsing, the word 'element' has been chosen in preference to 'activity'. This may have been because we have the idea of Four Elements in our own culture. Such a facile translation has led to a lot of misunderstanding because our conception of an element, from school days, is of a substance which, until the coming of atomic fission, could not be broken down into smaller parts. This is the very antithesis of the later use of the Wu Hsing, both in its philosophical and medical applications. The Five Activities of Water, Fire, Wood, Metal, Soil (Earth) are *processes*, in movement, and they interact. For instance, Water puts out Fire, Fire burns Wood, and so on.

Apart from this literal relationship, any activity which can be equated with Water, or placed in the same category as Water, tends to quell any Fiery type of activity. This is important as we try to understand everything in this chapter, because as Ted Kaptchuk points out, 'the common mistranslation of Five Elements . . . exemplifies the problems that arise from looking at things Chinese with a western frame of reference.'[16] We in the West tend to look for cause and effect; action number one produces result number two. The Five Activities do not so much cause something to happen as create a pattern in which something does happen. It is in their nature to be and act as they are. This has to be thought through many times, as far as I am concerned, before it even begins to sink in!

When the number Five is applied to certain phenomena it fits into it nicely, as for instance in the case of the four seasons. There are four seasons and the balance which exists between them makes up the number to five. Wood represents the state of things in growth, therefore Springtime; Fire the state of things which has reached maximum phase, and so Summer; Metal a declining state, Autumn, and Water a state of rest, Winter. Earth or Equilibrium is the natural balance between the four, the place where they inter-mingle but do not intrude upon one another.

The tendency to preserve and glorify the past, no matter what, led the proponents of the Wu Hsing into problems which can once more be illustrated by medicine. Below is a table showing the relationship given in medicine to Yin and Yang, Wu Hsing and organs of the body.

	Wood	Fire	Earth	Metal	Water
Yin organ	Liver	Heart	Spleen	Lungs	Kidneys
Yang organ	Gall bladder	Small intestine	Stomach	Large intestine	Bladder

The traditional relationships between the Five Activities and the organs, and those between the organs and the Yin-Yang concept were frequently at odds with one another. The Five Activities interpretation could say that the 'liver opens into the eyes' and the Yin-Yang that the 'chi of all organs is reflected in the eyes'.[16] Kaptchuk continues by saying the 'Five Phases (Activities) theory emphasises one to one correspondences, while Yin-Yang theory emphasises the need to understand the overall configuration upon which the part depends ... The Five Phases became a rigid system ... Yin-Yang theory ... with its emphasis on a Taoistic view of the importance of the whole, allowed for a great deal of flexibility.'

An interesting footnote as far as Tai Chi students are concerned is that neither Lao-tzu nor Chuang-tzu refer to the Five Activities, Phases or Elements, but they do refer to Yin-Yang theory. As quotations from both these sage sources are often cited by Tai Chi writers and teachers, this is significant.

This rigidity of the Five Activities theory has caused a lot of 'fudging' by the medical practitioners who have been determined to make it work in every case. From the moment the theory was written down, it was criticised.

In the Han dynasty a satirist wrote: 'The horse is connected with the sign wu (Fire); the rat with the sign tsai (Water); if Water really controls Fire, (it would be more convincing if) rats normally attacked horses and drove them away.' Here we come to the axis of any criticism of the Five Activities, especially in connection with our main interest, which is the interpretations given them by martial arts theorists. Kaptchuk gives the view that the Five Activities became 'entrenched' in the thinking of Chinese medicine because 'Chinese investigative study tends to be inductive only to a point and then proceeds with deductions based on the classics ... Most modern Chinese critics describe Five Phases theory as a rigid metaphysical overlay on the practical and flexible observations of Chinese medicine.'[16] This is reflected in the attitude of martial arts theorists.

The original name of Hsing-I Ch'uan could well have been Five Activities Boxing since its basic movements consist of five techniques. Pa-kua took its name from the Eight Trigrams, and Tai Chi from the diagram of the Supreme Ultimate. Tai Chi theory also takes the Eight trigrams and relates them to eight movements or gates and subdivided these into four directions and four corners.

☰	Ward Off	Sky	South
☷	Roll-Back	Earth	North
	Press	Water	West
	Push	Fire	East
	Elbow	Lake	Southeast
	Split	Thunder	Northeast
	Pull	Wind	Southwest
	Shoulder	Mountain	Northwest

The relationship of these movements to the directions and corners makes no sense at all from a logical point of view. The first four movements in the list of eight are all performed in roughly the same direction in forms. The eight movements do not have any logical relationship either with the meanings of the trigrams nor of the phenomena associated with them. The two exceptions are Ward Off and Roll-Back, Sky (Heaven) and Earth. Here the three Yang lines denote strong action which does relate to Ward Off, and the three weak lines of Roll-Back's trigram, Earth, denote yielding action. Attempts have been made to justify the six remaining movements with the meanings of the trigrams but they are very weak. For instance it has been said the movement Press is like water, because water gradually wears away the hardest stone by dripping. The movement of Push, Fire, has been described as very aggressive, like fire burning through a forest. But both of these things can be said about both of the movements willy-nilly, with the kind of associative arguments which are used by students in their appreciations of literature.

Other writers and teachers have taken this process even further and tried to relate Tai Chi to the hexagrams. If the process of relating movements to the trigrams was subjective and fanciful then that of relating them to the hexagram is even more so. A Tai Chi student may, over a long period, develop his or her own personal affinity with the I-Ching and connect its hexagrams with thoughts and feelings, imagination and sensations, but in my view this does not constitute a real, objective relationship at all.

Two versions of an interpretation of one of the hexagrams follows. Both will be seen to be valid. The process can be compared with a woman who goes to see a fortune teller. The fortune teller says that the woman is going to have news which will please her, but she may not recognise it as good news at first; that she must be alert also to her financial situation because if she is not she may run into difficulties; that there is a man she knows who thinks highly of her but something in her character is stopping him from saying so . . . These generalities are so general that they could be said with equal validity to any normal person, man or woman. They can be interpreted in dozens of ways, all equally possible. They do not represent telling the future at all. Similarly, the generalized meanings of the I-Ching cannot be applied to specific movements exclusively in any way which satisfies me, and I started off as someone who was quite happy to be a believer. The fact that a venerable, skilful and respected Tai Chi gentleman says that something in the I-Ching is related to a specific movement does not convince me. It is a case of 'one dog barks at a shadow and the rest bark at the sound'.

The hexagrams are approached in divination by dividing the six lines into two trigrams. This is the main and obvious division. Lines 4,5,6 make up the upper trigram and lines 1,2,3 the lower. Within the hexagram there are two that are called nuclear trigrams; the word nuclear having been chosen presumably because they lie inside, like a nucleus. The nuclear trigrams are taken from lines 2, 3, 4, 5 and overlap one another. Lines 2,3,4 make up the lower trigram and lines 3, 4, 5 the upper. This means that lines 3 and 4 are common to both though they have different places in each.

Having clarified for oneself the type of trigram according to the above method the first step is to look at what is called the Time. The category of Time gives the overall meaning of the hexagram: does it show increase or decrease, does it assist a process or cause conflict, how long will it last, and so on. The next category is called Place. This consists of examining each line, registering its position and its significance with regard to the other lines. There are other considerations, but this is enough to show that the interpretation of a hexagram is a complex subject. According to Wilhelm, 'Since the Han period . . . more and more mystery and finally more and more hocus-pocus have become attached to the book.' Though I may be shot down in flames for saying so I find that attempts to relate the hexagrams to Tai Chi movements does verge on 'hocus-pocus'.

INTERPRETATIONS

1. If we place the hexagram Ch'ien in front of a person performing the Tai Chi movement Ward Off Left and Ward Off Right in such a way that it is evenly spread, the fifth line is level with his jaw. When the left hand rises in Ward Off Left it reaches the level of the jaw, the fifth line. The existence of six strong lines in this hexagram evokes an image of strength and awakening, indeed of the stirring dragons mentioned in the I-Ching's interpretation of it. The second line's interpretation speaks of a 'dragon appearing in the field'. The field can represent the abdomen. If, in the next movement, of Ward Off Right, the rising hand goes too far, above the chin or fifth line, and reaches the sixth line, then according to the I-Ching an 'arrogant dragon will have cause to repent', meaning that the movement will look ugly and awkward.

This interpretation takes as its basis the position of the lines and the position of the hands in the movements concerned. In the case of the fifth line the hand position rising to the jaw is taken in a spatial sense, and the case of the second line is taken in a different sense altogether, because the second line is not level with the abdomen, but much further down. The idea of 'field' is found in some translations as the Tan T'ien, a point just below the navel, which is given in English as 'cinnabar field'. It can also mean earth.

2. If we take once more as our example the I-Ching's interpretation of the first line, which is 'hidden dragon, do not act' and say that this means that the lower legs and feet are filled with hidden power, ready to move when the time is right. The second line, 'dragon appearing in the field', means that the hidden power is projected into the whole body, or we could say into the Tan T'ien, cinnabar field, like celestial forces appearing on earth (field). The left hand rises like a dragon in the sky and the right hand settles down, towards the earth. This means that although the energy rises it is also at the same time rooted. One must beware of raising the left hand too high, to the sixth line, because this is the place of the 'arrogant dragon' and

an arrogant dragon opens itself to attack. The sixth line, being a Yang line at the end of a series of five Yang lines means that activity has reached its maximum and the only possibility is now to yield, return to Yin.

With a little imagination and ingenuity, combined with the right vocabulary, anyone can wander through the sixty-four hexagrams and produce highly plausible interpretations for all of them. Taking only the basic thirteen postures and the sixty-four hexagrams this would give us a total of a minimum of 832. If one then began to incorporate two, three or four hexagrams together then the number could rise to astronomic figures. At its best it seems that the I-Ching is a stimulus to thought and reflection about the possible movement inherent in Tai Chi, but direct and definitive interpretations are highly questionable.

It is in the application of Yin-Yang theory that Tai Chi finds its most helpful philosophical ally. As we saw in the chapter on postures we can give every posture-movement a predominantly Yin or Yang label. Advancing or retreating, shifting weight from one leg to the other making one leg full and the other one empty, can all be seen from a Yin-Yang standpoint. This is however only a superficial and obvious analysis. For instance in the movement of Roll-Back, student A pushes student B. In doing Roll-Back, B rests the inside of his right forearm on the outside of A's pushing left arm. B withdraws his body, retreating, Yin and diverts the push. Though B is retreating and yielding and so can be placed in the Yin category, he is also diverting so using a little Yang force. But as the Yang force of the diverting action is also making use of the Yin force of the whole retreating body it contains some Yang force. Furthermore, because B does not so to speak fly back or fall back like a stone in a vacuum, we can say that his overall yielding body action is supported by Yang acting as a brake, modifying the chief Yin movement.

By painstakingly and perhaps even a little pedantically analysing the directions and actions of B's body we find a whole network of Yin and Yang forces of varying degrees of strength all contained within the Yin of his Roll-Back. In order for this analysis to be valid, the movements themselves must be correctly performed, in a relaxed state, and with every muscle producing just the amount of energy needed. If for instance the shoulders and arms are unnecessarily tense and the legs not firm then the analysis which one could make for the ideal movement would no longer be valid.

Following in the footsteps of many other students of the Wu Hsing,

110

Five activities, Tai Chi practitioners have not been slow to find relationships. We looked earlier at the matter of difficulties which arose when this was done in the medical area and we find the same phenomenon in Tai Chi. One thesis which has been put forward is that there is a connection with five major organs of the body and five fundamental steps of the art: step forward, withdraw, look left, look right and balance. It is said that as each step is taken the student is promoting the health of a specific organ. It hardly seems necessary to say that this kind of claim cannot be taken seriously. To criticise it further would be like hitting an unconscious opponent.

Similar efforts have been made rotating the Five Activities themselves in a circle and connecting them with the five steps: water puts out fire. Five words were chosen and called the Five Words Secrets. Par excellence this demonstrates the taking of a revered idea from the past and fitting things in with it, no matter what the cost. As in the case of the I-Ching, endless arguments can be put forward to correlate the number five and Tai Chi. But the same can be achieved with three, four, six, seven, eight, nine as well. The idea of the Five Activities can be a stimulus and an intellectual basis for a beginner to start examining his movements. To try to fix oneself on that is a mistake.

What all three subjects of this chapter do is to provide an approach which Joseph Needham and Ted Kaptchuk, Richard Wilhelm and Iulian Shchutskii all wrote about in a positive way. They convey an idea of order and pattern to an art which is initially a difficult one for westerners to appreciate. It is in this respect that they can be most useful. When one tries to relate the I-Ching and the Five Activities to Tai Chi in detail, then that detail is not a help but a stumbling block.

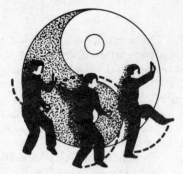

8 · TAI CHI POETRY

'Poetry in Motion' is the name of a song which was once popular in the West. A saying applied to the internal martial artist of China says, 'Looks like a Woman, Fights like a Tiger'. Training in the solo forms is certainly poetry in motion, and, equally, feminine on the outside but harbouring a tiger-like strength inside. When a student is able to do one of the forms in a satisfactory way, he or she experiences moods which can best be described as poetic, close to a religious experience. Then, analysis and comparison with systems of philosophy become unnecessary; as unnecessary as analysing the score of a piece of music by Mozart.

There are a number of classic Tai Chi poems praising the art and reminding students of its fundamental direction, but the chief work outside these specifically Tai Chi poems which is referred to in connection with the art is the *Tao Te Ching*. This book, par excellence an example of Fung Yu-lan's meaning of the word 'suggestive', has inspired millions of people in as many ways. Cheng Man-ch'ing gave talks to his students on the book, and gave them the advice, 'If sense and meaning collide, be content to suspend judgment'.[18] This might be taken as an instruction to the intellect when the *Tao Te Ching* is read and also when the Tai Chi forms are done. Once you can do a form, enjoy it, live it.

One of the telling verses of the *Tao Te Ching* begins, 'There is no single thing in all the world softer than water, more supple than water; yet in all the world is there anything to equal water in overcoming things which are hard and strong.' This theme is repeated in a later verse with, 'When a man is born he is soft and supple, but when he dies he is stiff and hard . . . That which is stiff and hard belongs to death, but the soft and supple belong to life.' The *Tao Te Ching* asks us if we can become soft and supple, like a child, breathing like a child, being permeated by breath but not 'stopping' the mind at breathing. These inspiring words can help to evoke in a student a kind of 'right' feeling about what he or she is doing. The movement of the Yang forms is continuous but should not become hard through the effort to be continuous. Students try to find a new rhythm in which continuity is not a strain, and breathing harmonises with this rhythm. The muscles and joints of the body respond to this and enjoy it. It seems for a while as if one has become a human being.

Throughout this book there is a kind of spirit which cannot be defined; something which, like continuous movement, loses its essential quality at soon as one attempts to pin it down; 'Tao follows the laws of its own nature.' To try to pin it down, define it, is to try to change its nature. This can be experienced when doing the forms of Tai Chi. I have already written too much about it!

Among the Tai Chi classics is an anonymous 'Song of the Thirteen Postures':

Keep the Thirteen Postures close; do not forget them.
When wishing to move, start from the waist.
Be sensitive to the changes, the slightest shift from full to empty.
Thus you let the Chi circulate like a flow through all your body,
    without ceasing.

Invisible in the embrace of stillness lies motion;
And within motion stillness is concealed.
Search, therefore, for that stillness within motion.
If you can approach this, discoveries will be yours when you meet
    your opponent.

Let every movement be filled with awareness and meaning.
If you can approach this, the effort of no effort will appear.
Never abandon your attention to your waist.
When the abdomen is light and free, the Chi will be aroused.
When the lowest vertebrae are upright, then the Spirit will rise to
    the top of the head.

The whole body should be pliant and soft,
The head suspended as if from above by a single hair.

Remain awake, searching for the meaning of Tai Chi itself.
Whether the body bends or stretches, whether it opens or closes,
Let the natural way be your way.
At the beginning, students listen to the words of their teacher,
But with care and effort they learn to apply themselves,
And then skill develops of its own accord.
Who can tell me, what is the main principle of Tai Chi?

The awakened mind comes first and the body will follow.
Who can tell me, what is the meaning and philosophy of Tai Chi?
Eternal youthfulness and a healthy long life, which mean
An ever present springtime.
Each and every word of this song is valuable and important to
    you;
If you do not listen to its words, and follow, you will surely sigh
    your life away.

Another, shorter instructional poem summarises the actions of Push
Hands. It is also anonymous and is simply called 'The Song of Push
Hands':

When you use the actions of
Ward Off, Roll-Back, Press and Push,
Let them always be filled with meaning.
When you move, remember that every part of the body is helped
    by another part.
If you move like this, no opening will appear
To let your opponent in.
If your opponent should use even the force of
One thousand pounds against you,
You can deflect it with the force of four ounces.
Lead your opponent into you; let him lose his own balance.
Combine yielding and attacking in one moment.

The famous Wang Tsung-yueh whom we met in the historical section
wrote an idealist description of Tai Chi mastery which is in a sense
poetic. It can be called poetic because the stages it describes can never
be reached by a human being; it is like a celebration of perfection in
the art. He says:

At the slightest pressure from an opponent, yield, and as soon as he
begins to retreat, stick to him . . . Match the speed of an opponent's
movements, by moving quickly when he does, and slowly when
he does. Whatever they may be, the multitude of techniques are

governed by the same principle ... Train with diligence and so move on to intrinsic energy and so move on to enlightenment ... Talent, intuition, things of this kind are not enough without long persevering effort. The brain should be clear and empty, and the Chi lowered to the Tan T'ien, with an upright, relaxed body. Any change in your balance should be hidden from your partner ... If you are pushed on your left side, it should be empty; If you are pushed on your right side, it should be empty. Wherever and whenever your opponent pushes you, he should find emptiness. As he comes forwards, your opponent should feel that he has leagues to go; as he goes backwards, he should feel hemmed in. If a feather drifted down on to your body, you would be so sensitive that you would feel it. If a fly were to settle upon you, you would be set in motion.

Such is the paragon of Tai Chi training, taking one's breath away with his awesome and untouchable skill; an inspiration if not a possibility. Wu Yu-seong, who changed from Yang to Chen style Tai Chi, also wrote about the art, along somewhat similar lines to Wang Tsung-yueh, but also speaking about the internal energies of the art. He had some striking similies.

Let your spirit be like a cat catching a mouse.
Let your manner be like a hawk stooping for a rabbit.
Let your stillness be that of a mountain.
Let your movement be that of a river.
Gathering together your Chi should be like drawing a bow.
Releasing your Chi should be like loosing an arrow.
Your mind is the general, your Chi the flag, your waist the flagpole.
When Ching moves, it should be like the reeling in of silk.

Other writers have tried to capture the spirit of Tai Chi in words but it is to these early works that students have turned time and again for guidance and a taste of the Supreme Ultimate.

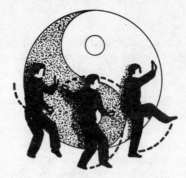

9 · HERBAL REMEDIES AND FOOD

It is a tradition in Chinese martial arts circles that a full-time instructor generally studies healing to a certain extent, so that he can help his students in case of injury when training. As far as Tai Chi Combat is concerned, injury can occur, but it is fairly rare, except in the case of the modern tournaments referred to earlier.

Wherever Chinese communities have been established, a herbal shop is sure to follow sooner or later. They all give off a marvellous smell which wafts out of the door into the street. Rows and rows of boxes fill the shelves, carefully labelled, or completely blank. On the counter are found clean sheets of paper piled up neatly beside a pair of scales. Outside one of the main London herbal centres there is always a queue to be found shortly before opening time. The customers file in, the assistants reach down the boxes, the contents are scooped out according to the prescription and wrapped up in the paper. Finally the contents of each packet is written in Chinese on the outside. This scene is I guess repeated the world over, because the Chinese people are great lovers of herbal remedies. Herbalism pre-dates acupuncture by several centuries.

Some Tai Chi and martial arts teachers have a second occupation as healers. A room is sometimes set aside behind the training hall and members of the public are greeted and treated there.

One of the commonest injuries is, of course, bruising. There is a common expression for the remedy for this – 'wine,' so named because rice wine of good quality is used as a base for it. Some 'wine' is drunk, to heal internal injuries and dissipate swelling, some 'wine' is applied to the bruise itself and some may be drunk and applied.

The best known eastern herb is of course ginseng, or *Panax Schinseng*, which belongs to the *Araliaceae* family. Although, it is not used for any of the physical injuries caused by martial arts, it is high on the Chinese list of generally-used herbs and has attracted a lot of attention in the West. It is a perennial herb and fetches a comparatively high price. In spite of the fact that many people swear by it, scientific tests on ginseng-taking in the United States have failed to produce any special results. But Chinese herbalists continue to insist that it will produce results such as increased metabolic rate, prevention of impotence, regulation of blood pressure and many other positive results.

Sir Edwin Arnold, the author of the book on the life of the Buddha, *The Light of Asia*, wrote of ginseng that 'It fills the heart with hilarity, whilst its occasional use will, it is said, add a decade to human life.' If this is so, we can all give up Tai Chi and take to drinking ginseng instead for our healthy longevity. Appealing to weight of numbers he goes on: 'Have all the millions of Orientals, all these many generations of men who boiled ginseng in silver kettles and praised heaven for its many benefits, been totally deceived?' One thing that several supporters of ginseng therapy say is that when it is part of a regimen ordinary Indian or Chinese tea should not be drunk. The word 'panax' comes from the same root as our 'panacea', meaning a cure for all things.

Did Professor Li Chung Yun live for two hundred and fifty years? If so, our quest for healthy longevity is solved again. In 1933 his death was announced in the New York Times. Chinese officials confirmed his age, saying that he had outlived twenty-three wives. In addition to taking herbs, a lifelong passion, it is reported that he also attributed his longevity to 'keeping a quiet heart, sitting like a tortoise, walking sprightly like a pigeon and sleeping like a dog'. Apparently Professor Li did not disclose all the names of his herbal remedies but two of them slipped out. One was our old friend ginseng and the other a less well known one called fo-ti-tieng. Unfortunately for readers of this book who want twenty-three wives or husbands and to live for two hundred and fifty years I do not know the botanical name fo-ti-tieng.

The urino-genital system of the body has always been a focal point for some Tai Chi theorists and the various occult groups and teachings which were mentioned earlier. Though I guess that the majority of Chinese men and women make love in more or less the same passionate way as the majority of the rest of the world population and their intercourse goes through the same stages, there seems to have always been somewhere in the offing a different attitude, kept relatively secret in the past but appearing from time to time in published books. Part of this secret was the idea that if men, and women, could merely enjoy intercourse and not come to a climax on every occasion, they would enjoy better health and live longer. It is part of the tradition of some Chinese martial arts to refrain from intercourse when training is severe, so that the 'vital essence', the Ching or essence of sperm, should not be dissipated.

Whatever the wisdom of these ideas, and others like them, any method which could promote health in the kidneys, bladder and sexual organs was always treated with respect, whatever modern science might say about it now. A number of herbs were looked upon as aids in this search for such health.

Our fo-ti-tieng is recommended in this respect, being good for the bladder. Juniper berries are used in teas, wines and oils for the kidneys and bladder, and since some types of back pain accompany disorders of the kidneys, juniper berries can also be said to be useful for relieving back pains. Other herbs for the kidneys and bladder are sage, marshmallow, clivers and parsley piert. (Readers are routinely advised not to act for themselves on any remedy given in this chapter but always to seek qualified advice.)

One of the plagues of the male reproductive system is enlargement of the prostate gland which presses on the urethra and prevents the passage of urine from the bladder. One of the herbs said to alleviate this complaint is parsley, prepared in the form of tea. In English we have our expression 'sowing his wild oats', referring to a young man's sexual adventures before marriage, so it may be no coincidence that the Chinese recommend an extract of oats in fluid form to tone up the sexual organs, especially after over-indulgence. Ginseng appears once again, in this group of herbs, though it is not the aphrodisiac which it is sometimes claimed to be. The more sober Chinese users say that by slowly building up the general health through regular use, ginseng can restore sexual functioning to a better level.

From the time of the Tang dynasty AD 618–907 herbalism became the predominant Chinese medical approach. Today there are far more Chinese physicians using herbs only to treat patients than there are ones using only acupuncture. The most recent pharmacopoeia lists 5,767 different herbs, minerals and animal extracts.[19] One should distinguish between what we can call folk medicine from traditional medicine. Many of the popular beliefs about ginseng, for instance, belong in the folk category. Traditional herbalism classifies herbs according to their uses, not according to their chemical content. Herbs also have a more specific and direct effect than acupuncture; the latter aims at the restoration of homoestasis rather than a specific cure. This means that herbs are more powerful and also can be more harmful if wrongly used. But it appears that there are a series of traditional checks on the use of herbs which makes wrong prescription difficult.

If a student of Tai Chi is training in order to improve health, then some acquaintance with Chinese herbal knowledge could be a useful adjunct to this. At the same time, since the wrong use of herbs can be harmful, it is advisable to find a good, reputable herbalist and not rely on self-prescription.

Over the last twenty years or so a new presentation of eastern approaches to food and health has spread thoughout the West in the form of the macrobiotic system. The chief promoter of macrobiotics has been the Japanese teacher, Michio Kushi. Though differing in many ways from traditional Chinese medical views, the basis of macrobiotics is said to be the ancient Yin-Yang Chia of philosophy. Since both the Chinese and macrobiotic systems are based on this ancient classification, the points on which they differ must be the result of a clash of interpretation. From its beginnings, macrobiotics centred on the understanding of food and drink and the classification of them into gradations of Yin and Yang. Then the sphere of its investigations extended into the worlds of exercise, acupressure, psychology and philosophy.

Here again the dangers of prescribing for oneself were evident when macrobiotics was a new craze, especially in the United States. Eating 'brown' or unpolished rice was one of the regular recommendations of macrobiotic specialists, as this particular food was seen as one which contained a balance of Yin and Yang qualities. Cases were reported of people putting themselves on a brown rice and water diet, and then suffering from malnutrition. From small beginnings, Michio Kushi[19] tried to re-present the Chinese classics with emphasis on Yin-Yang theory. On the philosophical level, statements such as 'Yin attracts Yang, Yang attracts Yin' were made in profusion. Various pieces of western scientific knowledge were listed to illustrate these statements. The eight trigrams and the sixty-four hexagrams were referred to and quotations from the Tao Te Ching and from religious teachers used, with the occasional questionable example: 'The teaching of Jesus was based on the same underlying principle called yin and yang in the Orient.'[19]

Kushi devoted some of his time and writing to the spiral shape and movement, which is found in Tai Chi. He pointed out that most of the galaxies of the known universe make a spiral shape, and on an infinitely smaller scale, that many phenomena such as sea shells are also constructed in spiral form. The DNA, which determines to a large extent what we are like when we grow up, takes a spiral shape and perhaps makes us think of Pre-Natal Chi and Pre-Natal Ching. Do they move in a spiral, and is Tai Chi echoing this spiral when one moves? By applying the polar theory of Yin and Yang to almost everything one could think of, Kushi produced a series of writings which are amazing in their variety whilst at the same time simple in their basis. Such an enterprise, to be thorough, is beyond the capacity of one man, and it will need careful study by his heirs and successors to develop and analyse his many statements before they receive scientific confirmation. What Kushi's tremendous undertaking does illustrate to students of Tai Chi is that of all the ideas from China's culture the Yin-Yang theory is the most helpful for an understanding of their art.

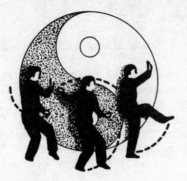

10 · TAI CHI AND BREATHING

Early in 1990 I started a beginners' class in Tai Chi and after a few minutes I asked the class if there were any questions. One woman, a complete beginner, said, 'What about breathing?' This was a fair question because the subject of breathing does appear in books on Tai Chi. In reply I said what I always say – that if we learn the forms, do them in a relaxed way and at an even tempo, then the breathing will take care of itself. This is my attitude, because it is the most natural. In the animal kingdom we find all kinds of movement and the movements of animals, birds, reptiles, fish and insects excel human movement in general. What animals have, and what we for the most part have lost, is the capacity not to interfere with their body movements. Tai Chi can be one of the things which helps us to undo that interference; to pile breathing exercises on top of the mess we have already made of ourselves is to load up with more problems.

An even more practical reason for leaving breathing exercises out of Tai Chi training is that it is difficult to learn the forms. If, as well as learning the forms, a student has to try synchronise his breathing, control his abdominal muscles and prolong or shorten the duration of inspiration and exhalation then he has even more to deal with.

The above is my advice, but since no survey of Tai Chi would be complete without outlining the approach taken by *some* teachers this chapter will look at their methods, in detail. My parting shot against such methods would be refer to Yang Cheng-fu's advice to

121

Cheng Man-ch'ing: relax, relax and then relax again, and everything else will follow.

The role of the breath in the functioning of human beings has been documented for centuries, in China, India, Japan and other countries. This documentation was always related to specific disciplines such as the cure of illness, training in Indian Yoga, the Taoist religion's search for immortality and so on. If a person is not ill, does not want to become an Indian Yogi or find immortality then it could be argued that the exercises described in books are not anything to do with him or her.

In addition to such sources, one cannot help noticing the part breathing plays in ordinary daily life. When my three children were little, and occasionally burst into tears, I discovered a simple way of stopping their crying if it seemed to be going on for too long. I would ask them to blow their noses, because without fail if they had a good blow then the crying stopped. In time, one by one they spotted the connection between blowing the nose and stopping crying and sometimes they would refuse to blow because they knew they would have to part company with their grievance as soon as they did so, and grievances can be very dear to a child's heart. Everyone has heard the expression, 'Take a deep breath' – this is part of our common folk lore for people who are going to do something difficult.

An inscription on a piece of jade from the Chou dynasty 1027–256 BC speaks about holding the breath, the expansion of the breath, the solidification of the breath and the movement of the breath.[20] Most of the references to breathing in subsequent writings relate it to the Tan T'ien, the spot just below the navel, in which it is said that Chi can be stored. The role of the breath in this storing of Chi was to assist the mind in bringing the Chi to this point. If the Chi could be so stored then the theory is that this can lead to further psychic possibilities.

Modern research into such theories has not gone very far, but one finding, which is connected with theories about the anaesthetic effects of acupuncture, was the discovery of endorphins. Endorphin is a substance which calms down the organism and helps it to eliminate fear, as well as sensations of pain. Exactly how it works is not known, as far as I am aware. It is, however, clear from research that one of the effects of heroin is to stimulate the flow of endorphin. It is likely that one of the reasons for the calming effects of deeper breathing over a prolonged period is that endorphin is produced in greater quantities when the organism is breathing in this way.

One of several modern researchers into breathing therapy is Tadashi Nakamura, a professor of clinical psychology of the Oriental

Respiratory Research Institute. He was attracted to the study of breathing as a therapeutic method after graduating from the Sociology Department of Meiji Gakuin University in Japan in 1962. His research led him to study Primal Scream Therapy.[20] He also noted the use of deep breathing exercises to help veterans of the Vietnam war to recover from some of the deep traumas they had suffered in combat duty, and the increasing attention given to breathing methods by many members of the medical profession all over the world. With these and other pieces of evidence from the scientific quarter he turned to investigate what he could of the older traditions of breathing therapy and then attempted a correlation of the two. A summary of what he has to say would be a helpful way of re-presenting the kind of breathing methods used in some Tai Chi training, as it will eliminate the obscure references and figurative language which clouds this tradition.

Nakamura began by showing that the relationship between breathing and emotional states is a clearly established fact. When a person moves from a depressed to a happy frame of mind the diaphragm movement increases and the expansion of the lungs likewise. In an experiment, some people depressed about their difficult financial circumstances were given the suggestion that they had found some large sums of money lying in the street. Automatically the diaphragm and lungs responded as anticipated. Further simple collation of existing data showed that lung function peaks in the majority of people around the age of twenty and that by the age of sixty it has reduced to the level of a nine year old. We can therefore appreciate that regular Tai Chi training, inducing deep and relaxed breathing, may well counteract some of the effects of ageing. Without special athletic training or physical work, the quantity of air breathed in can be as little as 400 cc and with such training and work can increase to 3,500 cc.

The regulatory mechanism for breathing in the human nervous system is located in the medulla oblongata, near the occiput, where the skull meets the vertebrae of the spine. The insistence in Tai Chi training and in the Alexander system on the importance of the head's relationship to the spine is connected to this. Good head-spine posture and good muscle tone of the region contributes to improved breathing. When Zen monks sit for long periods in meditation the position of the head and spine plays an important role in the deep abdominal breathing which they follow. Tests showed that even though a Zen monk may breathe between only two and five times a minute, without strain, and a normal breathing rate may be say eighteen times a minute, the number of litres of air inhaled and exhaled will be the same.

After a number of further experiments and comparison with the data of other workers in the field, Nakamura summarised the results of deeper breathing on the digestive organs, the circulation and the nervous system. In doing so he confirmed the claims which have been made for some years, but in the more poetic language of the Chinese culture, by Tai Chi teachers. Prolonged deeper breathing stimulates the stomach, liver, kidneys and intestines. A simple but welcome effect is to relieve constipation. It also assists in the absorption of nourishing substances by the digestive organs by affecting the capillary vessels, and promotes excretion by the kidneys. The circulation system is assisted by deep breathing because it helps prevent the accumulation of cholesterol and stimulates the activity of the red and white blood corpuscles. The absorption of oxygen and the elimination of carbon dioxide proceeds more efficiently.

The division of the nervous system into sympathetic and para-sympathic, stimulation and sedation, is regulated by deep breathing and in this respect Nakamura cites the presence of Ki (the Japanese word for Chi). Ki, he maintains, is assisted in its work by better functioning of the respiratory system. At this point Nakamura departs from his strict reliance on western scientific methods and the use of statistical analysis and returns to the beliefs of his fathers . . .

Having laid down his proofs of the benefits of such breathing, he goes on to present a number of cautionary words about the use of breathing exercises. Here he makes a clear distinction between normal, healthy people and people who are unwell. Speaking of the latter, he says, 'Once under control (the breathing) they should endeavour to continue natural breathing'.[20] Among the effects of deep breathing therapy, which can be adverse unless properly supervised, are dizziness and pain, variations in heart beat, temporary diminishing of the sense of taste, abnormal itching of the skin, wind, loosening of the bowels, nocturnal emissions and feelings of heaviness. People with arteriosclerosis and hypertension should be especially careful with breathing exercises. Nakamura also touches on the use of visualisation of the benefits expected from breathing therapy, a method used by holistic therapy centres. He likens this to bringing together the Ki and the 'I' (ee), the Chinese word for mind.

The ideal standing posture for breathing therapy is similar to that used by Kenichi Sawai of the Tai-ki-ken style of martial arts, feet apart a little wider than the hips and the arms held in a horizontal 'circle' level with the shoulders. In this posture a process is supposed to take place which is the same as the one found in the Chinese Tai Chi tradition. The Ki 'condenses' at the Tan T'ien, under the influence of the 'I' and the breath, and rises to the top of the head through the spine and also down to the tips of the toes.

As far as the exact location of the Tan T'ien is concerned, Nakamura quotes various 'old books' and gives four different locations. One is nine centimetres below the navel, another between the kidneys and the navel itself, a third some four centimetres below the navel, and the fourth at the intersection of two acupuncture channels; one running round the waist and the other running down the front of the body. It is tempting to choose the last location because the Chinese character for T'ien, *field*, is like a rectangle with a vertical cross in it, and one feels that this crossing point could be related to the crossing of the two channels. Maybe in this case we should resist temptation and simply say that the Tan T'ien is near the navel and probably below it.

The main idea in the beginning stage of this therapy is that during breathing one tries to bring the attention down to the Tan T'ien in order to feel free from thoughts in the brain. Nakamura quotes a saying that 'attention protects the Tanden' [29] (Japanese for Tan T'ien). He explains a further benefit of focusing on the Tan T'ien by pointing out that it is near the solar plexus, a part of the nervous system whose tension is part of many undesirable emotional states. Just like most Tai Chi teachers and students, Nakamura focuses almost all of his thinking on the Air Chi which we mentioned earlier, and apparently overlooks the Pre-natal and Grain Chi, speaking of Chi as if it were all one type of energy, like water in a tap, and as if human beings were like a plumbing system, with water being accumulated, pumped and sprayed throughout it. Also, despite his earlier warnings in his book he says quite irresponsible things such as 'take the Ki into yourself slowly through the nose by breathing and contain the Ki inside your body. You must then count in your mind up to the number 120 and then respirate the breath through your mouth slowly.' Making a practice of holding the breath for two minutes or more is not advisable and is just the kind of thing to avoid when doing exercise and Tai Chi training. He then really goes to town on this idea quoting an ancient text which says that 'you have to repeat the breathing practice until you count to 1,000 in your mind'. By that time all your troubles will be over because you will be dead – sixteen and a half minutes! – unless of course you are a Yogi . . .

Leaving aside the last two examples, Nakamura tries to present some of the breathing lore of the East in conjunction with western findings, and in doing so confirms some traditional Tai Chi beliefs.

The methods he puts forward are therapeutic, not for normal healthy people. Secondly he uses the mind to directly change the breathing, by counting, holding the breath and visualising in conjunction with this. The approach suggested by Yang Cheng-fu on the other hand uses the mind to relax the body first, then the breath follows this relaxation; this seems preferable and less likely to cause harm.

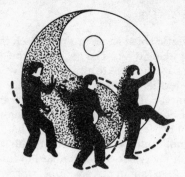

11 · TAI CHI TODAY

Since I first started Tai Chi, some time in 1968, the spread of the art throughout the world has been amazing. At that time there were few westerners who had even heard of it, let alone seen it. As far as I know there were only two people teaching the art in London and one of them was a visiting American. I leave aside the many Chinese who were possibly practising on their own and out of sight. Just over twenty years later every evening institute has its Tai Chi teacher and many colleges have Tai Chi clubs. In addition there are plenty of private clubs and independent teachers, as well as regular visiting Chinese teachers from the United States, Taiwan, China, Singapore and Malaysia.

The main style taught has been the Yang style, but in recent years the Chen style has come up, along with styles synthesised by the Chinese athletic organisations. Push Hands is becoming more widespread and Tai Chi Combat is getting a hold in various forms. Sadly, Pa-kua and Hsing-I have not shared in this rise in popularity.

Many clubs insist that the students wear the traditional Chinese outfit for training, consisting of a jacket fastened by braid toggles and a Mandarin collar. Others allow casual clothes. The two most important points about clothing are the trousers and shoes. Trousers should allow freedom of movement, jeans are out, and shoes should give the foot a comfortable flat surface on which to rest so that there is no danger of over-balancing. Trainers with thick soles are a menace in this respect. They may be all right for jogging but not for Tai Chi.

The rubber or plastic soled Kung fu shoe which is very popular with students I do not like, myself. The impact on the ground is very dead and some of them are inclined to slip. I usually wear a pair of very old and comfortable leather shoes with a rubber sole.

Prices charged for Tai Chi lessons vary very much. Evening institutes are the cheapest but in private clubs one can pay as much as £5.00 or £7.50 per lesson. But private teachers have overheads to meet which do not apply to institutions in the same way. It is also true to say that in many cases the standard of tuition in institutions is not always equal to that in private clubs, where the teacher is often full time and has a long background in martial arts. Many evening institutes have teachers who would not rate at all in martial arts circles. However this is probably true in many other subjects as well as Tai Chi, and provided a teacher can do a form passably well, why not learn from him or her.

In my experience, the fact that someone can do Tai Chi well does not mean that he is also a qualified historian, philosophy master, doctor, athletic coaching specialist or expert Taoist mystic. When one is in a pupil-teacher relationship with someone, one's critical faculties may be blunted. If the teacher says something about Tai Chi which is perfectly accurate and true, then in the same sentence says something about medicine, history or philosophy, one might make some reservations about the second half. As I hope this book has made clear, the world of Tai Chi today is like an enormous warehouse in which the past has accumulated. If a student wishes to understand it he must start sorting it out for himself.

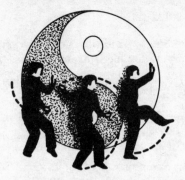

BIBLIOGRAPHY

1. Fung Yu-Lan, Professor   *A Short History of Chinese Philosophy*, Macmillan, 1948.

2. *Tao Te Ching, trans.* C. H. Ta-Kao, Unwin, 1976.

3. *Chen Style Taiji Quan, compiled by* Zhaohua Publishing House, Beijing, 1984.

4. Cheng Man-Ching   *Master Cheng's Thirteen Chapters on T'ai Chi Ch'uan, trans.* Douglas Wile, Sweet Ch'i Press, 1982.

5. Smith, R. W.   *Chinese Boxing, Masters and Methods*, Kodansha, 1974.

6. Suzuki, D. T.   *Zen and Japanese Culture*, Princeton University Press, 1973.

7. Chen, Yearning K.   *Tai Chi Sword, Sabre and Staff, trans.* Stuart Alve Olson, Bubbling Well Press, 1986.

8. Ju-Pai, Dr Tseng   *Tai Chi Weapons*, Paul H. Crompton Ltd., 1982.

9. Sawai, Kenichi   *Taiki-Ken*, Japan Publications Inc., 1976.

10. Stevens, John   *Abundant Peace*, Shambhala, 1987.

11. Chung-yan, Chang   *Creativity and Taoism*, Wildwood House, 1975.

12. Shchutskii, I. K.   *Researches on the I-Ching*, Routledge, 1980.

13. *Sources of Chinese Tradition* Volume 1, *compiled by* William Theodore De Bary, Columbia University Press, 1960.

14. Needham, Joseph   *Science and Civilisation in China* Volume 2, Cambridge University Press, 1956.

15. *I-Ching, trans.* Richard Wilhelm, Routledge, 1965.

16. Kaptchuk, T.   *Chinese Medicine: The Web That Has No Weaver,* Rider, 1983.

17. The *Yellow Emperor's Book of Internal Medicine, trans.* Ilsa Veith, University of California Press, 1972.

18. Cheng, Man-Jan   *Lao Tzu: My Words Are Very Easy To Understand*, North Atlantic Books, 1981.

19. Kushi, Michio   *The Book of Macrobiotics*, Japan Publications Inc., 1977.

20. Nakamura, Tadashi   *Oriental Breathing Therapy*, Japan Publications Inc., 1977.

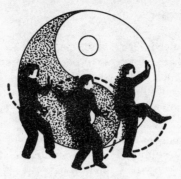

GLOSSARY

Aikido – A Japanese martial art employing body movements which in some instances resemble those of Push Hands of Tai Chi.

The Art of War – A seminal book of uncertain date containing ideas on warfare which probably influenced all forms of Chinese martial arts (Sun Tzu, *trans*. Thomas Cleary, Shambhala Publications 1988).

Blood – A term used in traditional Chinese medicine to describe not only blood in the Western sense but also various functions which it carries out.

Ch'an Buddhism – A form of Buddhism peculiar to China, emphasising direct experience of reality rather than thought, and based on a blending of Taoism and Buddhism.

Chen – The name of the family which produced the Chen style of Tai Chi; more varied in speed, posture and combative application than any of the other styles.

Chi – Vital energy, intrinsic energy, vitality which accompanies the activities of all life.

Chi Kung (Qi Gong) – The art and science of cultivating the Chi in human beings; currently prominent in the treatment of sick people in China.

Ching (Jing) – A vital energy recognised by traditional Chinese medicine and directly related to the growth and development of human beings.

Five Animals – An ancient form of Chi Kung using the imitated movements of animals, for example: tiger, deer, bear, monkey, crane, to promote health and longevity.

Five Elements – Earth, fire, water, metal and wood, these represent five phases through which all processes are supposed to pass; a complex and at times controversial idea.

Fluids – The most 'Yin' of all the substances in the human body recognised by Chinese traditional medicine. They include urine, sweat and saliva.

Form – The sequences of unbroken movement used in Tai Chi to exercise the body, study the postures and cultivate the Chi.

Hsing–I – One of the three major internal martial arts of China. It uses an extensive range of animal movements and is the most vigorous of the three.

I–Ching – An ancient book of divination, with extensive commentaries and interpretations which has influenced Chinese culture profoundly.

Nei-Chia – An expression meaning 'internal school' (of martial arts) which has sometimes been used, probably erroneously, to describe Tai Chi.

Pakua (Bagua) – An expression meaning 'eight trigrams'. In martial arts it refers to a form of combat and training supposedly based on the symbols found in the I-Ching. One of the three major internal martials arts of China.

Posture – A misleading term suggesting a static pose in the Tai Chi Forms. In reality the 'postures' are simply distinct movements found in a Form.

Push Hands – A two person exercise used in Tai Chi training to develop a sense of the inter-play of Yin and Yang, yielding and pushing.

Shen – The finest energy in human beings according to traditional Chinese medicine. It has been translated as 'spirit'.

Sun – A style of Tai Chi invented by Sun Lu-T'ang; now almost extinct.

Taiki-Ken – The Japanese rendering of Tai Chi Chuan and also the name of a style of combat taught in Japan based on the internal martial arts of China.

Taoism – A form of Chinese philosophy and self cultivation.

"Tao te Ching" – A book of Taoist wisdom, popularly attributed to the sage Lao-tzu, but more likely a compilation of writings from various sources.

Trigram – An arrangement of three parallel broken or unbroken lines denoting Yin or Yang energy, combined in pairs to form the hexagrams (six lines) of the I-Ching.

Wu – The name of the family which produced the Wu style of Tai Chi.

Wushu – An expression meaning 'martial arts' and generally preferred by purists to the better known western usage of the word Kung-fu.

Yang – The name of the family which produced the Yang style of Tai Chi which is today the best known outside China.

Yin-Yang – A fundamental division of forces into opposites: female-male, dark-light, yielding-aggressive. The name of a school of Chinese philosophy.

Zen – Ch'an Buddhism was introduced to Japan over a period of time, it took root and was developed along Japanese lines and known as Zen Buddhism.

INDEX